Evidence-Based Teaching
Current Research
in Nursing Education

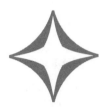

NLN PRESS SERIES

Evidence-Based Teaching
Current Research
in Nursing Education

Kathleen R. Stevens, RN, EdD, FAAN
Editor

Virginia R. Cassidy, RN, EdD
Associate Editor

JONES AND BARTLETT PUBLISHERS
Sudbury, Massachusetts
BOSTON   TORONTO   LONDON   SINGAPORE

World Headquarters
Jones and Bartlett Publishers
40 Tall Pine Drive
Sudbury, MA 01776
978-443-5000
info@jbpub.com
www.jbpub.com

Jones and Bartlett Publishers Canada
2406 Nikanna Rd.
Mississauga, Ontario
Canada L5C 2WG

Jones and Bartlett Publishers International
Barb House, Barb Mews
London W6 7PA
UK

PRODUCTION CREDITS
SENIOR EDITOR   Greg Vis
PRODUCTION EDITOR   Linda S. DeBruyn
MANUFACTURING BUYER   Kristen Guevara
TEXT DESIGN   Argosy
EDITORIAL PRODUCTION SERVICE   Argosy
TYPESETTING   Argosy
COVER DESIGN   Anne Spencer
PRINTING AND BINDING   Braun-Brumfield

Library of Congress Cataloging-in-Publication Data
Evidence based teaching : current research in nursing education /
    Kathleen R. Stevens, editor ; Virginia R. Cassidy, associate editor.
        p.   cm.
    At head of title: NLN Press.
    Includes bibliographical references and index.
    ISBN 0-7637-0937-9
    1. Nursing—Study and teaching—Miscellanea.   2. Nursing—Study
and teaching—Research—Miscellanea.   3. Evidence-based medicine—
Study and teaching.   I. Stevens, Kathleen R.   II. Cassidy,
Virginia.   III. National League for Nursing.
    [DNLM: 1. Education, Nursing.   WY 18 E935 1999]
RT73.E94   1999
610.73'071—dc21
DNLM/DLC
for Library of Congress   99-11150
                                                               CIP

Printed in the United States of America
02 01 00 99   10 9 8 7 6 5 4 3 2

Contents

Preface

Research is fundamental to excellence in the preparation of nurses. To this end, the Council for Research in Nursing Education (CRNE) of the National League for Nursing (NLN) and Jones & Bartlett Publishers present *Evidence-Based Teaching: Current Research in Nursing Education.*

Evidence-Based Teaching evolved from a solid basis of dissemination of education research, established through 12 years of publication of the series, *Review of Research in Nursing Education. Evidence-Based Teaching* reflects its ancestry by presenting summaries and analyses of educational research literature on specific topics. Through this dissemination of research, the CRNE wishes to influence faculty, students, and programs to strive for maximum efficacy and relevance to the profession and to health care.

The goal of *Evidence-Based Teaching* is to improve nursing education practices and programs by providing a scholarly basis. This publication inaugurates an expansion to meet growing needs for scholarly discussions about nursing education. Chapters approach discussions through (a) summarizing existing science on educational strategies and innovations, emphasizing implications of the science; (b) providing a scholarly discussion of issues affecting students, teachers, faculty, administrators, nursing education, and its research; or (c) developing a collective of analytical wisdom about educational models.

Also in keeping with the goal of dissemination, the entire series *Evidence-Based Teaching* is indexed in the Cumulative Index to Nursing and Allied Health Literature (CINAHL). We hope that these expansions will contribute to the scholarship of teaching and appeal to our readership as nursing education continues its metamorphosis into the twenty-first century.

Evidence-Based Teaching presents a variety of topics essential to progressive nursing education. The first chapter advances the concept of evidence-based nursing education, trends in nursing education research, and the crucial nature of integrative reviews of literature in the evolution of education. The second chapter describes mentorship in all levels of nursing education as an important element in subsequent professional success and satisfaction. In the third chapter, research on the essential process of teaching psychomotor nursing skills is reviewed. The fourth chapter explores a particular ethical issue in higher education—academic dishonesty, a troublesome issue of prime importance to those concerned with the integrity of education programs and with stewardship of the socially mandated role of the nurse. The fifth chapter updates the research evidence in predicting success on state board licensure examination. Reflective of the current trend in health care, the sixth chapter reviews educational preparation of nurse practitioners as advanced-practice nurses. The seventh chapter is also an update and suggests implications for graduate curricula from the utilization patterns of the graduates of master's and doctoral programs.

The volume is a collective work of authors who sought to share their analyses with our readership. Their commitment to excellence has been evident throughout the publishing process, and their discussions are recommended to nurse faculty and students of professional education. These research-based discussions will surely enhance our educational endeavors. Many thanks are extended to these authors, as they have made this volume possible.

Each chapter underwent careful peer review by members of the Editorial Review Board. These board members generously shared their expertise during the review process and provided valuable guidance, for which both the editors and the authors are thankful.

It is our sincere wish that the efforts invested in this volume culminate in continued scholarship and excellence in nursing education.

Kathleen R. Stevens, RN, EdD, FAAN
Editor

Virginia R. Cassidy, RN, EdD
Associate Editor

Chapters Contained in Past Volumes of *Review of Research in Nursing Education*

Volume 7

- Models of Nursing Education for the 21st Century
- Role Strain, Roll Stress, and Anxiety in Nursing Faculty and Students
- The Significance of Student-Faculty Interactions: A Review of the Literature
- Research on Teaching in the Clinical Setting
- Spirituality and Nursing Education
- Utilization of Master's and Doctoral Program Graduates: Implications for Curricula
- Predicting Success on the Registered Nurse Licensure Examination: Past, Present, and Future

Volume 6

- Teaching and Learning at a Distance: A Review of the Nursing Literature
- Caring: Curricular Issues
- Doctoral Education in Nursing: A Comprehensive Review of the Research and Theoretical Literature
- Empathy: Theory, Research, and Nursing Applications
- Retention of Nursing Students: Intervention Strategies

Volume 5

- Review of Research on Critical Thinking in Nursing Education
- Nontraditional Students in Higher Education: A Review of the Literature and Implications for Nursing Education
- Qualitative Research in Nursing Education
- Nursing Research Related to Educational Re-Entry for the Registered Nurse
- A Review of Literature on Changing Answers on Multiple-Choice Examinations

Volume 4

- Retention/Attrition of Nursing Students: Emphasis on Disadvantaged and Minority Students
- Review of Research on Male Nursing Students
- Preceptorship in Nursing Service and Education
- Review of Research Literature Related to HIV Diseases: Implications for Nursing Education
- Research on Values and Values Education
- Research on Prelicensure Nursing Education in Canada: Progress, Promise, and Problems

Volume 3

- Research on Teaching Methods
- Moral and Ethical Development Research in Nursing Education
- A Review of Literature on Mentor–Protégé Relationships
- Review of Research on Creative Problem Solving in Nursing
- Research on the Differences Between Baccalaureate and Associate Degree Nurses
- The History of Research in Public Health Nursing Education

Volume 2

- Learning Styles: Theory and Use as a Basis for Instruction
- Clinical Judgment: A Comparison of Theoretical Perspectives
- Administrative Leadership and Faculty Scholarship: Research on Nursing Faculty and Deans
- Video and Computers in Instructional Media Research
- Evaluation in Staff Development Education
- Mandatory Continuing Education: A Review of the Empirical Evidence
- ERIC: A Resource for Researchers in Nursing Education

Volume 1

Part One: Nursing Education in the Academic Setting
- Research on Clinical Judgment
- Professional Socialization of the Registered Nurse
- Research on Clinical Teaching
- Predicting Academic Success
- Stress of the Returning RN Student

Part Two: Nursing Education in the Service Setting
- Stress and Critical Care Nursing
- Research Studies in Hospital Staff Development
- The Clinical Nurse Specialist

Editorial Review Board

Joan Thiele, PhD, RN
Professor of Nursing
Intercollegiate Center for Nursing
    Education
Washington State University
College of Nursing
Spokane, WA 99204

Theresa M. Valiga, EdD, RN
Dean, College of Nursing
Fairfield University
North Benson Road
Fairfield, CT 06430-5195

Valvyne M. Viers, PhD, RN, CS
6301 Thirlmare Ct.
Austin, TX 78754

Mary Boose Walker, EdD, RN
Assistant Dean for Graduate Studies
School of Nursing
Widener University
Chester, PA 19013

Sue Young, PhD, RN
School of Nursing
Widener University
Chester, PA 19013

Contributing Authors

Patricia Bailey, EdD, RN
Professor of Nursing
University of Scranton
Department of Nursing
Scranton, PA 18510

Martha J. Bradshaw, RN, PhD
Associate Professor
School of Nursing
Medical College of Georgia
Augusta, GA 30912

Dona Rinaldi Carpenter, EdD, RN
Associate Professor of Nursing
University of Scranton
Department of Nursing
Scranton, PA 18510

Betsy Frank, RN, PhD
Professor
School of Nursing
Indiana State University
Terre Haute, IN 47809

Judith Fullerton, CNM, PhD, FACNM
Professor, College of Nursing and
    Health Sciences
University of Texas at El Paso
El Paso, TX 79902

Colleen Keller, RN, C, PhD
Professor
The University of Texas Health Science
    Center at San Antonio
San Antonio, TX 78284

Arlene Lowenstein, RN, PhD
Director, Graduate Programs in Nursing
MGH Institute for Health Professions
Boston, MA 02114

Donna Jo Miracle, RN, C, MSN
Assistant Professor
Anderson University
Anderson, IN 46012

Roberta K. Olson, PhD, RN
Dean and Professor
South Dakota State University College
    of Nursing
Brookings, SD 57007

Kathleen R. Stevens, RN, EdD, FAAN
Professor
The University of Texas Health Science
    Center at San Antonio
San Antonio, TX 78284

Connie Vance, EdD, RN, FAAN
Dean and Professor
College of New Rochelle School of
    Nursing
New Rochelle, NY 10805

Chapter 1

Advancing Evidence-Based Teaching

KATHLEEN R. STEVENS, RN, EDD, FAAN

INTRODUCTION

Nursing education research has not yet been fully synthesized, and evidence-based guidelines for teaching are in the early stages of development. Just as clinical research informs clinical nursing practice, nursing education research informs educational practice. The future of our profession lies in effective, efficient, and visionary preparation of our clinicians. In today's practice-focused climate, nurses must remember that teaching is a scientifically based practice.

The *raison d'être* for research in a practice discipline is to provide scientific guidelines for effective and efficient practice. So it is in the practice of nursing and the practice of nursing education. Nursing education should be efficient (for both teacher and learner) and should produce intended educational outcomes. Although knowledge produced through research provides stable and valid evidence to support decision making related to practice, a gap remains between nursing education research and nursing education practice. The purpose of this chapter is to advance the concept of evidence-based practice to evidence-based teaching. The following aspects will be discussed: (a) basic terms and processes of evidence-based practice, (b) availability of nursing education research as requisite to utilization of research in practice, and (c) future directions for evidence-based teaching.

DEFINITIONS

The use of research results to guide nursing practice has been called *research utilization* or *research-based practice*. A recent trend in medical and health care research (also influencing nursing) has generated the term *evidence-based practice*. In this vein, the term *evidence-based teaching* is advanced in this discussion. Each of these terms implies using research-generated knowledge to improve practice and its outcomes.

Such terms as *review of literature, integrative review of research, evidence synthesis, systematic review, knowledge synthesis, meta-analysis,* and *synthesis of science* have been used to describe variations or aspects of this process. Each term refers to systematic review processes undertaken to reduce a number of sources of research knowledge into a coherent summary of the science. In this discussion, synthesis of science is taken as the broadest term, inclusive of the other terms.

Research utilization is defined as "the use of knowledge generated through research to guide nursing practice" (Burns & Grove, 1997, p. 797). An earlier definition of the term identified it as "basing the practice, education, and management of nursing on research findings" (Stetler, 1985, p. 40). The history of research utilization has been chronicled in other sources (e.g., Burns & Grove, 1997; Stetler, 1985); however, Stetler's specific inclusion of education in the definition of research utilization is notable.

Evidence-based practice is a method of problem solving that involves identifying a clinical problem, searching the literature, evaluating the research evidence, and deciding on the intervention (White, 1997). It is derived from the term *evidence-based medicine,* which is the "conscientious, explicit and judicious use of current best evidence in making decisions about the care of individual patients" (Sackett, Rosenberg, Gray, Haynes, & Richardson, 1996, p. 1). In this very young trend, the term has been expanded to evidence-based health care, and evidence-based nursing; each term implies the use of research results in interactions with the client, care decisions, and, more broadly, practice.

Extrapolating from the definitions above, this discussion advances a definition of evidence-based teaching to be "the conscientious, explicit, and judicious use of current best evidence in making decisions about the education of professional nurses." Another, simpler definition is that evidence-based teaching is "the use of knowledge generated through research to guide nursing education practices." Evidence-based teaching includes the arenas of teaching, learning, curriculum development, and education administration.

BASIC STEPS IN DEVELOPING EVIDENCE-BASED PRACTICE

Evidence-based practice is a new paradigm, as is the process of developing evidence-based practice. Bringing research to bear on practice can be outlined in four fundamental steps:

1. A sufficient body of research on the phenomena of interest must exist; relevant phenomena must be investigated through the conduct of research.
2. The research must be identified and synthesized into a meaningful body of knowledge.
3. Synthesized evidence must be translated into models or analogues that guide practice decisions and actions.
4. The evidence-based practice must be implemented and evaluated within the organizational context of the practice.

In this way, the research of nursing develops knowledge that informs practice.

To provide the most relevant and effective nursing education, nurse educators must incorporate the essence of this evidence-based practice movement into nursing education as evidence-based teaching.

CATALYSTS FOR DEVELOPMENT OF EVIDENCE-BASED PRACTICE

The larger context of health care greatly influences nursing education, as does the context of higher education. In health care, a growing demand for justification of health care interventions and care systems has arisen from the public and from policymakers. The demand has been to evaluate interventions and related outcomes in terms of improvement in patients' lives and cost of care (Hinshaw, 1992). Such an emphasis has spurred the momentum of outcomes research, incorporating evaluation methods, epidemiology, and economic theory (Burns & Grove, 1997). Nursing's response to this demand is seen in development of research application, research utilization, and research-based practice models. (See, for example, Titler et al., 1994, and Goode & Titler, 1996, describing the Iowa Model for Research in Practice.) The evidence-based practice trend has gained momentum, producing evidence-based practice guidelines, best practice recommendations, and an acceleration in efforts to develop evidence synthesis methods.

Similarly, in higher education, calls for "application scholarship" (Boyer, 1990) emphasize the public demand for relevancy and pragmatism in education outcomes. In 1990, a movement to reexamine scholarship was launched by Boyer (1990). These concepts also apply to teaching, which Boyer viewed as "the highest form of understanding" (1990, p. 23). He placed teaching "at the very heart of the scholarly endeavor. Teaching is also a dynamic endeavor involving building bridges between the teacher's understanding and student's learning. Pedagogical procedures must be carefully planned, continuously examined, and relate directly to the subject taught" (1990, p. 24). This continuous examination of pedagogy in nursing education can be accomplished through research to discover effective, efficient means of teaching and correlates of learning.

Following Boyer's redefinition of scholarship, the wide-scale reexamination of research in academic settings broadened traditional views of scholarship-as-research. Scholarship was expanded to include scholarship of discovery (research), scholarship of integration, scholarship of teaching and learning, and scholarship of practice. Prior to this, other fields such as engineering and medicine separated discovery and practice, emphasizing academic rewards for research. By virtue of the applied nature of research in nursing (research to solve problems), scholarship in nursing education had not followed the traditional academic model. The prevailing academic model was basic research—producing knowledge for the sake of knowledge (Boyer, 1990). Nursing faculty roles maintained pragmatic application of research scholarship because nursing developed from a client-centered practice. Faculty, therefore, bore responsibility for the entire range of intellectual endeavors, from research to implementation in practice to educating new clinicians (Rice & Richlin, 1993). Although the academic value system of nursing has always been tempered with pragmatism, this movement for reexamination of scholarship provided an opportunity for academic formalization of a core value in nursing: applied research.

VALUE OF RESEARCH TO PRACTICE

The value of research-based practice in nursing is clear. One synthesis of 84 nursing intervention research studies demonstrated that research-based nursing interventions produced a 28% improvement in client outcomes over traditional nursing interventions (Heater, Becker, & Olson, 1988). This result was evident in a similar summary of research studies on the effects of nursing interventions on children and parents (Olson, Heater, & Becker, 1990).

Indeed, Hancock (1996) stated, "The development of evidence-based practice has to be among the most important developments in health care today. If we are to place a true value on the care that nursing provides, we have to understand that value in terms of effectiveness and not just in terms of cost. And if we are to make meaningful decisions about which services are purchased and provided in future, we have to know which treatments work and why" (p. 20). Surely, the value of research-based nursing education practices parallels that of clinical practice.

In spite of the demonstrated and intuitive appeal of improving practice through research, nurses have encountered barriers to achieving this goal. Some of the major barriers to research utilization noted by clinicians were related to characteristics of the individual using the research, characteristics of the organization or setting in which the research was to be implemented, the qualities of the research, and the communication of research knowledge. Related to communication, the following specific barriers were identified: complexity of statistical analysis, scattered literature, unclear practice implications, unclear research report, and nonrelevance to practice (Funk, Tornquist, & Champagne, 1995). One approach for addressing these barriers is synthesis work, such as systematic reviews. Systematic reviews directly address all of these problems in communicating research knowledge, rendering it highly usable by the clinician or educator. A systematic review "repackages" a collection of research studies such that the knowledge and implications for practice are clearly communicated. This approach can also be effective in the educational arena. Placing such education research reviews in the hands of educators who wish to incorporate research knowledge into their teaching practices, pedagogy, and processes will remove many of the barriers to research utilization and will facilitate evidence-based teaching.

AVAILABILITY OF NURSING EDUCATION RESEARCH

To develop evidence-based teaching, there must exist a body of completed research studies that investigate phenomena of interest to nursing education. Some of these core phenomena are teaching strategies, learning processes, learner characteristics, learning outcomes, academic success, effects of technology mediation, organization of curriculum, workforce development, theory verification, measurement and methodological issues, educational program standards, and administrative effectiveness. To determine whether a critical mass of nursing education research exists, we can examine general trends in nursing research and current status of nursing education research.

Trends in Nursing Research

Trends in nursing research have followed the profession's transition into the academic setting and attendant focus on scientific scholarship. These trends are evident in both the focus of the research and the number of studies conducted.

The focus of research can be described by the proportion of research conducted on educational topics and on clinical topics. Indeed, this proportional emphasis of nursing research is reflected in a number of sources. In the years immediately following the American Nurses Association's 1964 position statement on educational preparation, nursing research focused on human resources necessary to meet this challenge: faculty preparation, characteristics of nurses and students, and academic programming (Downs & Fleming, 1979). In fact, from 1957 to 1982, nursing research predominantly focused on clinician preparation rather than on clinical research.

This trend was apparent in three separate assessments of nursing research during this time. In 1957, Henderson reviewed the then-meager collection of nursing research studies and developed a classification system for nursing research (Henderson, 1957). A second assessment was conducted by Abdallah (1970), who classified 167 U.S. Public Health Service grants and found that 93% of the studies focused on health workforce, care systems, nurses' roles, and faculty development, while the remaining 7% were classified as clinical research. Abdallah (1970) concluded that nurses tended to investigate educational and administrative issues rather than clinical practice issues. In 1982, a third assessment of research substantiated that 91% of nursing research studies investigated professional and educational issues and 9% investigated clinical phenomena (Walker, 1982). During the developmental phase of nursing from 1970 to 1982, the proportion of research on educational and professional issues far exceeded the proportion of clinical research, as depicted in Figure 1–1.

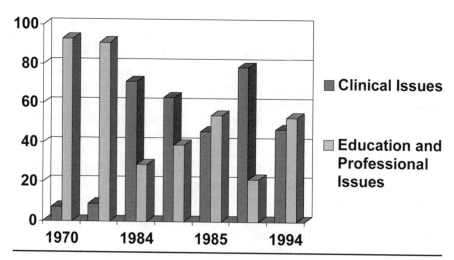

FIGURE 1–1.
Trend in Emphasis of Nursing Research, 1970–1994

In the mid-1980s, research began to focus on clinical issues. The new clinical emphasis reflected nursing's dedication to improving nursing care effectiveness; however, nursing education research was left in the wake. Most research studies conducted during the mid-1980s were classified as clinical research studies, as verified by three separate assessments. One assessment of cancer nursing research (Fernsler, Holcombe, & Pulliam, 1984) clearly showed the shift in research emphasis, with 29% of the research studies classified as educational and professional issues research and 71% classified as clinical research. Another assessment of nursing science (Brown, Tanner, & Padrick, 1984) verified this shift of emphasis in the broader scope of nursing research, concluding that 37% of the studies focused on educational and professional issues whereas 63% of the studies focused on clinical issues. A third assessment categorized 54% of the reviewed studies as educational and professional issues research and 46% of the studies as clinical research (Jacobson & Meininger, 1985). A review of doctoral dissertations from nursing schools from 1976 to 1982 also confirmed the trend, indicating that only 22% of the dissertation studies were educational and professional issues research, whereas 78% were clinical studies (Loomis, 1985).

To examine the trend toward clinical research and away from education research, Stevens (1994) assessed dissertations in the 1994 Cumulative Index to Nursing and Allied Health Literature (CINAHL) bibliographic database (Stevens, 1994). (Note that only dissertations from 1988, 1989, 1990, and 1991 were fully indexed in CINAHL at that time.) These dissertations ($N = 2,227$) were sampled using interval sampling with a random start to select a minimum of 100 data elements for analysis. The resulting sample of dissertations ($n = 115$) were then classified according to primary topical area into one of four categories: clinical, nurse characteristics, nursing education, and health care system. Table 1–1 shows that 19% of the dissertations focused on nursing education topics, whereas 47% focused on clinical topics (Stevens, 1994).

These results indicate that dissertation research remained primarily focused on clinical topics during the 10 years following Loomis's 1985 examination. Following Loomis's forecasting logic that dissertation research represents the research of the future decade, it was concluded that the proportional emphasis

TABLE 1–1.
Classification of a Random Sample of Dissertation Topics, 1988–1991

Topic of Study	Number	Percent
Clinical	54	47
Nurse characteristics	29	25
Nursing education	22	19
Health care system	10	9
TOTAL	115	100

on education research studies through the end of the century was likely to remain low. Moreover, the trend was likely to continue because it had been institutionalized by the formation of the National Institute for Nursing Research (NINR, originally National Center for Nursing Research) in 1986: The research priorities of NINR are clinical in nature, supporting basic and clinical nursing investigation (NINR, 1993).

Trends in Nursing Education Research

This overview indicates that, regardless of the classification taxonomy and groupings used for these research studies, since 1982 the shift from educational research toward clinical research has been dramatic and sustained. This trend in nursing studies clearly reflects the profession's primary social responsibility for direct clinical care and its fundamental need for research to inform clinical practice. Unfortunately, this shift expressed itself as a decrease in the proportional emphasis on nursing education research.

After noting that the bulk of nursing research had migrated to clinical issues in 1984, nurse researchers were cautioned: Research regarding nurse characteristics, nursing education, and nursing administration should not be completely abandoned, in that those factors profoundly affect the type and quality of care nurses deliver (Brown et al., 1984, p. 31). The value of scientifically based education and administrative practices was underscored.

Although the proportional emphasis of research has shifted away from nursing education topics, nursing education research studies are still being conducted. Another approach in examining this trend is to estimate the number of education research studies being conducted. The major journals that publish nursing education literature are *Journal of Continuing Education in Nursing, Journal of Nursing Education, Journal of Nursing Staff Development, Nurse Educator,* and *Nursing and Health Care* (Swanson, McCloskey, & Bodensteiner, 1991). Each journal publishes nursing education research reports, albeit at various rates or proportions of the total number of articles published (see Table 1–2). Using the total number of articles published and the proportion of these articles that are research reports, the number of research articles was estimated for the years 1993 to 1997. This estimate shows that almost 2,000 nursing education research reports were reported in these five journals over five years.

A second approach to examining the trend in nursing education research is to compare the number of studies published per year over three different time periods. To do this, findings from Loomis (1985) and Stevens (1994), and the estimates reported in Table 1–2 were used to calculate the number of nursing education research studies conducted per year from 4- to 5-year periods from 1976 to 1997. Table 1–3 compares the volume and yearly rates for the three time periods.

The trends show a decrease in the proportion of education research studies being conducted, accompanied by an increase in the number of education

TABLE 1–2.
Estimated Number of Nursing Education Research Articles Published in Five Major Nursing Education Journals, 1993–1997

Journal	Number of Articles Published[1]	Research Proportion[2] (%)	Estimated Number of Research Articles
Journal of Continuing Education in Nursing	812	50	406
Journal of Nursing Education	1,401	80	1,121
Journal of Nursing Staff Development	692	10	69
Nurse Educator	1,040	10	104
Nursing and Health Care	875	30	263
TOTAL			1,963

[1] As indexed in CINAHL, 1983–1997.
[2] From Swanson, McCloskey, & Bodensteiner (1991).

TABLE 1–3.
Comparison of Volume of Education Research in Three Time Periods

Time Period	Total Number of Education Research Studies	Yearly Rate (Number of Studies per Year)
1976–1982 (Loomis, 1985)	70	70 studies/6 years = 12 studies per year
1988–1991 (Stevens, 1994)	423	423 studies/4 years = 105 per year
1993–1997 (see CINAHL search above)	1, 963	1,963/5 years = 393 per year

research studies. This numeric increase confirms that phenomena of interest to nurse educators are being investigated. A numerically large body of research on these phenomena is being produced, generating a corpus of evidence to guide education practice. This body of research is the requisite component in the development of evidence-based teaching.

SYNTHESIZING SCIENCE

Once a body of research is generated, the second step in developing evidence-based teaching is to synthesize research on given topics; however, complications arise when there is more than one research study or when the results are incongruous (Kavale, 1995). Synthesis of a number of research reports into a coherent body of science is a complex undertaking in light of variations in design and analysis and in the event of contradictory findings. This task is particularly difficult in behavioral sciences because these sciences rarely demonstrate linear progress and development (Kavale, 1995). The need for systematic research synthesis is further emphasized by the escalating volume of studies published yearly in virtually every scientific field, including nursing education science.

Types of Systematic Reviews

A systematic review is "the process of systematically locating, appraising, and synthesizing evidence from scientific studies in order to obtain a reliable overview. Systematic reviews are distinct from traditional literature reviews in that they are based on a strict scientific design. Often literature reviews are based on only a selection of published literature and reflect the views of the reviewers. Systematic reviews are comprehensive, following a scientific design in order to minimize bias, and ensure reliability" (National Health Services Centre, 1996, p. 4). Methods for systematic reviews have been detailed in a number of disciplines. Some of these methodological discussions are found in the sources identified in Table 1–4.

This table shows that science can be synthesized through a number of methods. These summaries are accomplished for two major reasons: to identify the gaps in knowledge, and to identify the existence of knowledge. When the intended activity is to conduct research, the primary objective of the summary is to identify what is not known (gaps in knowledge), setting the stage for the proposed research. When the intended activity is to develop evidence-based practice, the primary objective of summarizing science is to identify what is known. This seemingly minor shift in the paradigm of summarizing science creates a major shift for nursing education researchers and educators. The intense focus on developing nursing research within academic settings has led to an almost singular scientific mission of identifying gaps in knowledge to validate the need for research. The advent of evidence-based teaching now swings the mission to affecting education practices with what is known. Consequences include an increased accountability for educational outcomes and an increased need to access and translate education research results into educational practices.

Demonstrating Value of Systematic Reviews

While the rigor of systematic reviews is somewhat daunting, their value is clear. The generalizability and validity of conclusions from a systematic review far

TABLE 1–4.
Summarizing Science: Sources of Methodological Discussions of Various Types of Systematic Reviews

Type of Systematic Review	Source	Description
Literature review	Burns & Grove (1997)	Analyzes and summarizes research to define what is known and not known about a topic.
Integrative review of literature	Cooper & Hedges (1994)	Integrates empirical research to create generalizations; includes statistical meta-analysis and integrates theory, resolves conflict, and identifies central issues for future research.
Meta-analysis	Hunt (1997)	Merges numerical results from a number of studies, discovering consistencies over the studies.
Systematic review	Berry (1996)	Locates, evaluates, and synthesizes scientific studies using strict scientific design; the aim is to ensure a comprehensive and unbiased review.
	Mulrow & Oxman (1994)	Consists of a clearly formulated question that uses systematic and explicit methods to identify, select, and critically appraise relevant research, and to collect and analyze data from the studies included in the review. Statistical methods (meta-analysis) may or may not be used to analyze and summarize the results of the included studies.
Knowledge synthesis	Sigma Theta Tau International (STTI) (1993)	Summarizes research-based knowledge on a topic; includes annotated bibliography of key studies and practice implications.

exceed those of a single study. In addition, the "investment of science" in the studies represented in a systematic review is much greater than the investment in a single study. A simplistic quantification of the value of a summary of research studies (systematic review, traditional review of literature, meta-analysis, or other) can be expressed using Stevens' Index of Science-Years (published for the first time in this manuscript). This index demonstrates one facet of the value of a published systematic review of research—that of investment in terms of years.

Stevens' Index of Science-Years

Stevens' Index for Science-Years referenced in a given review articles is

Minimum completion time (3) × number of studies cited = science-years

© Stevens 1997

The index is based on the assumption that a typical research study requires a minimum of 3 years to complete (from conception through implementation, reporting, and publication). Calculating science-years represented in a single systematic review may increase one's appreciation of the science represented in that review. By comparison, the number of science-years represented by a single research study is far less than that represented in a systematic review. While this simple approach does not assess the rigor of a systematic review, it expresses the value of the review in terms of total investment of time to produce the science.

Rigor of Systematic Review Methods

Systematic review methodology is relatively new and has only recently been examined for rigor. In assessing the state of the science of review articles, Mulrow (1987) examined medical review articles, concluding that reviewers did not, at that time, routinely use scientific methods to identify, assess, and synthesize information. However, since that time, systematic methodology has further developed, as evidenced by the Cochrane review method (Mulrow & Oxman, 1994) and integrative literature review approach (Cooper & Hedges, 1994). As the use of systematic review methods increases in nursing, nurses will be able to analyze the rigor of the review.

Prevalence of Systematic Reviews

How prevalent are systematic reviews in nursing? Semantic difficulty exists when identifying published systematic reviews because of the variety of terms used to label and index the reviews in bibliographic databases. The following overlapping terms are commonly used in indexing systematic reviews: review of literature, research-based nursing practice, evidence-based practice, integrative review of literature, and meta-analysis.

To estimate the prevalence of summaries of science in the nursing literature, an automated search of the 1998 CINAHL bibliographic database was performed. Each term was individually searched, and article type was limited to research. Although "review of literature" is commonly the least rigorous approach to systematic review, it is included here as a reference point in nursing literature. The numbers of articles for each type of systematic review are presented in Table 1–5. A total of 160 systematic reviews of nursing research were located, showing that systematic review is a relatively new approach in synthesizing nursing science.

Meta-analysis as Systematic Review

To examine meta-analysis as a specific type of systematic review, this category was further analyzed. The fundamental goals of meta-analysis are to combine results across individual studies to yield an overall estimate of effect for the purpose of integrating the findings (Glass, 1976). Although the relatively short history of meta-analysis has been fraught with controversy (Hunt, 1997), it has emerged as a new scientific discipline that is expected to endure. Indeed, Chalmers (1994) commented that "this series of techniques of combining published and unpublished data from multiple research projects has such striking advantages over the classic review article that it should largely replace the latter in the medical literature" (p. 1).

The search showed that, prior to 1987, no meta-analytic study was indexed in CINAHL. During the 5 years from 1988 to 1992, 19 meta-analytic studies were published. During the next 5 years, another 52 meta-analytic studies were published, bringing the total to 81 meta-analyses. This search located only two meta-

TABLE 1–5.
Number of Articles Indexed as Systematic Reviews in CINAHL

Search Term	Number of Articles
Review of literature[1]	1,218
Research-based nursing practice (limited to review articles)	71
Integrative review of literature	8
Meta-analysis	81
Total number of systematic reviews (excluding reviews of literature)	160

[1] Provided as a reference.

analytic studies on topics in nursing education. The first summarized differences in performances of baccalaureate, associate degree, and diploma nurses (Johnson, 1988); the second meta-analysis summarized the research comparing computer-based instruction with other educational strategies (Cohen & Dacanay, 1994).

As a specialized method of systematic review, meta-analysis is extremely underutilized in nursing education research. This is attributable, in part, to the descriptive and correlational nature of educational research and, in part, to the low use rate of meta-analysis in nursing in general. In general, systematic review methodologies are designed to synthesize randomized control trials. Specialized methodology for systematic reviews of descriptive, correlational, and qualitative research would make possible synthesis of a larger portion of nursing research, yet such methodological development is in its infancy.

PUBLICATIONS FOR SYSTEMATIC REVIEWS IN NURSING EDUCATION

To what extent is the corpus of nursing education research systematically reviewed? This question may be partially answered by considering the success of one source of literature reviews: *Review of Research in Nursing Education*. Sponsored by the National League for Nursing Council for Research in Nursing Education, this series presents systematic reviews of educational research. The goal of the series is to improve nursing education practices through application of research. Begun in 1986, the *Review* has published summaries and critical analyses of educational research literature on various topics. Each chapter contains a review of research, a summary of science on a specific nursing education topic, and recommendations for education practices. Reviews have been published on such topics as clinical teaching, distance education, computer-mediated teaching, critical thinking, clinical judgment, moral and ethical development, and mentorship. To date, a total of 50 chapters have been published in the *Review* series. Publication of such reviews have significantly contributed to the scientific basis for teaching, however, the additional rigor of systematic review methods would provide even stronger bases to guide education practices.

STRATEGIES FOR THE FUTURE

Strategies for advancing evidence-based teaching in the immediate future can be identified. One is to increase the corpus of nursing education research, thus providing a basis for evidence-based teaching. A second is to disseminate education research widely, and a third is to develop a national research agenda for nursing education. Each of these strategies is discussed in further detail below.

Increase the Corpus of Nursing Education Research

A great need exists for increasing the number and expanding the type of nursing education research studies. This is because both nursing and nursing education continue to change, producing a need for research on new phenomena that assume priority for nurse educators. Among these new phenomena are community-based education, practice-based education, critical thinking, expanded roles in nursing, specification and evaluation of learning outcomes, technology-mediated teaching and learning strategies, and distance education. A specific example is the advent of technology, which has provided the ability to greatly extend distance education (distributive education) far beyond the single dimension of paper-based correspondence courses. As technology-mediated strategies develop, the mandate to examine strategy effectiveness is incumbent on the nurse educator.

Indeed, the new environments for education and practice are creating opportunities for the development of new approaches to teaching and the concomitant scientific evidence of effectiveness. Nursing education researchers must redouble their efforts in educational research to ensure the preferred future for nursing education—one in which education programs are evidence-based; are contemporary in strategy, form, and content; and have predictable learner outcomes.

Notwithstanding the obvious need for such research, there is a shortage of resources for nursing education research. Although human and fiscal resources to support nursing education research are minimal, this barrier can be overcome. This critical shortage requires that nursing education researchers be creative in capturing resources to use in studies. Several approaches for finding resources can be suggested. First, through examining educational settings and strategies, nursing education researchers may be able to capitalize on "natural experiments." Changes and revisions in health professions education and health care delivery produce natural experiments and provide opportunity for investigation requiring few additional resources. Such natural experiments might include comparing outcomes of learning activities pre- and postchange; comparing acceptability and impact of technology-mediated educational strategies; and correlating distributed education (distance education) with learner outcomes.

Another major strategy for conducting significant research with few resources is to append research questions to larger scale systematic program evaluation. Similar to the natural experiments described above, program evaluation differs in its broader scope of potential impact. Program accreditation bodies mandate evaluation of many phenomena that are also of interest to nursing education researchers, so education program evaluation has much to offer nursing education research. Program evaluation views an education program as a system of interrelated components designed to produce specific outcomes (Stufflebeam & Webster, 1994), such as a graduate nurse prepared to function within a variety of dynamic health care environments. Moreover, systematic program evaluation holds an advantage over single-study evaluation of instructional methods in improving education practices. Program evaluations are typically comprehensive, evaluating a broad spectrum of program elements (e.g., context, resources, processes, and outcomes), and are often linked to continuous program improvement (Cavanaugh, 1993). Experts have also recommended ways to develop theoretical frameworks for educational program evaluation (Bourke and Ihrke, 1998). In addition to these direct links to program improvement, program evaluation studies should be planned with the explicit purpose of contributing to the understanding of phenomena (Stufflebeam & Shinkfield, 1985). In this way, program evaluation contributes to research activities. Indeed, sophisticated evaluations can provide "partial probes of theoretical ideas" (Shadish, Cook, & Leviton, 1991, p. 9). Program evaluation promotes scholarly efforts to understand education practice because program evaluation has evolved into a process based on theory.

Another approach to furthering education research is to develop automated information systems that archive education program information not only for program evaluation and administrative use but for research use as well. Such systems would facilitate secondary data analysis of educational phenomena from archived information. This analysis of archived data has several benefits. Archived information is a relatively inexpensive data source for research analysis, and it is useful in generating hypotheses for further research, comparing findings from different studies, and examining trends (Graves, 1998b).

An obvious prerequisite to secondary analysis in nursing education is the existence of a database. To maximize the usefulness of education databases over time and across programs, the underlying classification schema of the database must be standardized, much as the minimum data set for clinical nursing has been developed (see Werley & Lang, 1988). As computer-based student and curriculum records are developed, a standardized data classification schema should be developed to accommodate future research. Although no direct recommendations for doing this are currently available, the principles learned from development of clinical information systems (e.g., Zielstorff, Jette, & Barnett, 1990) and from management data sets (Huber, Schumacher, & Delaney, 1997) can guide education research database development. Databases that can be mined for research data regarding student performance, progress, and characteristics as well as program variables would greatly enhance secondary analysis in education research. Databases that can be placed in data set repositories for secondary analysis would establish not only a basis for comparison but also a means to explore research questions.

Following the logic of Werley and associates (Werley, Devine, Zorn, Ryan, & Westra, 1991; Werley & Lang, 1988), a nursing education minimum data set must be formed. As this data set is developed, nursing education researchers must establish its research utility (see Delaney, Mehmert, Prophet, & Crossley, 1994). At present, there is no concerted national effort to achieve this objective. Structures underlying accreditation reviews could provide a beginning structure for development of a minimum nursing education data set.

Disseminate Education Research Widely

To maximize the impact of nursing education research, the findings must be widely disseminated. Currently, a number of excellent nursing education journals disseminate research reports; describe new instructional methods, education theory, and concepts; and discuss issues. As researchers study natural experiments, perform secondary analysis of existing data sets, and conduct program evaluation research, the results must be published to contribute to the body of evidence guiding practice. Existing journals should be used to disseminate these research studies; however, new formats and outlets are needed to facilitate dissemination. These include technology-mediated education research conferences, capturing the conference proceedings for a wider audience. Additionally, systematic reviews should be aggressively developed to synthesize education research into efficient education guidelines.

Beyond publication of single research study reports, systematic reviews of nursing education research should be conducted and widely disseminated. While a number of journals publish single research reports, currently only three publishing channels routinely publish systematic reviews: *Review of Research in Nursing Education, Annual Review of Nursing Research,* and *Online Journal of Knowledge Synthesis for Nursing. Review of Research in Nursing Education* (described earlier) is solely dedicated to the publishing integrative reviews of nursing education research. *Annual Review of Nursing Research* includes systematic reviews on clinical, educational, administrative, and professional issues. *Online Journal of Knowledge Synthesis for Nursing* publishes systematic reviews via the World Wide Web. While the *Online Journal* has published only reviews of clinical topics in nursing to date (e.g., deep vein thrombosis prevention in surgical patients, courage in chronic illness, and weaning from mechanical ventilation), recent plans include expansion to nursing education topics (Jane Barnsteiner, editor of *Online Journal of Knowledge Synthesis for Nursing,* personal communication, December 4, 1998). Nursing educators can use these publication channels to disseminate systematic reviews and as resources to advance evidence-based teaching.

An additional channel for dissemination of nursing education research is the Registry of Nursing Research. The registry is housed in the Sigma Theta Tau International (STTI) Nursing Library and is a resource for researchers and students (STTI, 1998). The registry, provided to advance all types of scholarship in nursing, was planned to accommodate nursing education research along with clinical and other domains (Graves, 1996). This unique electronic registry is a database of researcher biographical data, project information, and research results. Automated searches of this database can be performed using research concept, variable name, keyword, researcher's name, or researcher's institution. Two main features make this registry unique:

1. Both published and unpublished studies are included.
2. Study information is classified into a tailor-made classification system, the Nursing Research Classification System (Graves, 1998c).

As education researchers begin studies, registering their projects, even during the conduct of the research, will help build a network among education researchers. Once results are available, these are placed in the registry in a unique form: variable by variable, with the findings indicated. This will be the basis for synthesis of knowledge using a knowledge engineering program called *arcs©* (Graves, 1998a). In the near future, *arcs©* will provide automated assistance in synthesizing research findings across a number of research studies. It produces computational modeling of the research knowledge by using "scientific findings reported in research literature as data with which to propose theoretical models" (Graves, 1998a, p. 353).

Priorities for Nursing Education Research

Consensus was established for priorities for nursing education research in 1987 (Tanner & Lindeman, 1987). Using the Delphi technique with nurse educators, Tanner and Lindeman rank ordered critical research questions regarding nursing education. Priorities for research included the following topics: integration of research findings into nursing curricula, development of problem-solving skills, approaches to clinical teaching, and level of practice of graduates of different basic preparations.

Events in health care, the curriculum revolution, and the surge of technology have greatly affected nursing education and presumably nursing education research priorities. In the more than ten years that have passed since Tanner and Lindemann's study, new issues have arisen, including community-based education, practice-based education, critical thinking, expanded roles in nursing, globilization of nursing, specification and evaluation of learning outcomes, technology-mediated teaching and learning strategies, and distance education. Which of these topics is in most immediate need of investigation? Given the events of the last decade, the education research agenda set forth by Tanner and Lindeman (1987) is in need of reexamination. Recently, the National League for Nursing Council for Research in Nursing Education established a blue ribbon panel to reconsider nursing education research priorities. These revised priorities will be consequential as resources are allocated for activities that contribute to educational excellence in nursing.

CONCLUSIONS

The trend toward evidence-based practice holds promise for improving nursing education practices. Advanced here is the concept of evidence-based teaching accompanied by a number of strategies to move nursing education toward using research evidence as the scientific basis for educational practices.

REFERENCES

Abdallah, F. G. (1970). Overview of nursing research 1955–1968: Part I. *Nursing Research, 19,* 6–17.

American Nurses Association. (1965). *A position paper: Educational preparation for nurse practitioners and assistants to nurses.* Kansas City, KS: American Nurses Association.

Berry, L. (1996). The systematic literature review: What it is and how it can help: An interactive primer. (Available: http://agora.leeds.ac.uk/comir/people/eberry/sysrev/sysrev.htm.)

Bourke, M. P., & Ihrke, B. A. (1998). The evaluation process: An overview. In D. M. Billings & J. A. Halstead (Eds.), *Teaching in Nursing*. Philadelphia: Saunders.

Boyer, E. L. (1990). *Scholarship reconsidered: Priorities for the professoriate.* Princeton, NJ: Carnegie Foundation for the Advancement of Teaching.

Brown, J. S., Tanner, C. A., & Padrick, K. P. (1984). Nursing's search for scientific knowledge. *Nursing Research, 33*(1), 26–32.

Burns, N., & Grove, S. K. (1997). *The practice of nursing research* (3rd ed.). Philadelphia: Saunders.

Cavanaugh, S. H. (1993). Connecting education and practice. In L. Curry & J. F. Wergin (Eds.), *Educating professionals: Responding to new expectations for competence and accountability,* pp. 104–126. San Francisco: Jossey-Bass.

Chalmers, T. C. (1994). Implications of meta-analysis: Need for a new generation of randomized control trials. In K. A. McCormick, S. R. Moore, & R. A. Siegel (Eds.), *Clinical practice guideline development: Methodology perspectives* (AHCPR Publication No. 95-0009, pp. 1–3).Washington, DC: U.S. Department of Health and Human Services.

Cohen, P. A. & Dacanay, L. S. (1994). A meta-analysis of computer-based instruction in nursing education. *Computers in Nursing, 12*(2), 89–97.

Cooper, H., & Hedges, L. V. (Eds.) (1994). *The handbook of research.* New York: Russell Sage Foundation.

Delaney, C., Mehmert, M., Prophet, C., & Crossley, J. (1994). Establishment of research utility of Nursing Minimum Data Set. In S. J. Grobe (Ed.), *Proceedings of the Fifth International Conference on Nursing Use of Computers and Information Science* (pp. 163–168). San Antonio, TX: International Medical Informatics Association.

Downs, F. S., & Fleming, W. J. (1979). *Issues in nursing research.* New York: Appleton-Century-Crofts.

Fernsler, J., Holcombe, J., & Pulliam, L. (1984). A survey of cancer nursing research January 1975–June 1982. *Oncology Nursing Forum, 11*(4), 46–52.

Funk, S. G., Tornquist, E. M., & Champagne, M. T. (1995). Barriers and facilitators of research utilization: An integrative review. *Nursing Clinics of North America, 30*(3), 395–407.

Glass, G. V. (1976). Primary, secondary, and meta-analysis. *Educational Researcher, 5,* 3–8.

Goode C. J., & Titler, M. G. (1996). Research for practice. Moving research-based practice throughout the health care system. *MEDSURG Nursing, 5*(5), 380–383.

Graves, J. R. (1996, Second Quarter). New classification system announced. *Reflections,* pp. 24–28.

Graves, J. R. (1998a). Representation of knowledge for computational modeling in nursing: The *arcs©* program. In J. J. Fitzpatrick (Ed.), *Encyclopedia of nursing research.* New York: Springer.

Graves, J. R. (1998b). Secondary data analysis. In J. J. Fitzpatrick (Ed.), *Encyclopedia of nursing research.* New York: Springer.

Graves, J. R. (1998c). The Sigma Theta Tau International nursing research classification system. In J. J. Fitzpatrick (Ed.), *Encyclopedia of nursing research.* New York: Springer.

Hancock C. (1996). Proving nursing works. *Nursing Standard, 11*(3), 20.

Heater, B. S., Becker, A. M., & Olson, R. K. (1988). Nursing interventions and patient outcomes: A meta-analysis of studies. *Nursing Research, 37*(5), 303–307.

Henderson, V. (1957). An overview of nursing research. *Nursing Research, 6,* 61–71.

Hinshaw, A. S. (1992, October). Welcome: Patient outcome research conference. In *Patient outcomes research: Examining the effectiveness of nursing practice* (proceedings of a conference sponsored by the National Center for Nursing Research, September 11–13, 1991 (NIH Publication No. 93-3411). Washington, DC: U.S. Department of Health and Human Services, Public Health Services, National Institutes of Health.

Huber, D., Schumacher, L., & Delaney, C. (1997). Nursing management minimum data set (NMMDS). *Journal of Nursing Administration, 27*(4), 42–48.

Hunt, M. (1997). *How science takes stock: The story of meta-analysis.* New York: Russell Sage Foundation.

Jacobson, B. S., & Meininger, J. C. (1985). The designs and methods of published nursing research: 1956–1983. *Nursing Research, 34,* 306–312.

Johnson, J. H. (1988). Differences in the performances of baccalaureate, associate degree, and diploma nurses: A meta-analysis. *Research in Nursing & Health, 11*(3), 183–197.

Kavale, K. A. (1995). Meta-analysis at 20: Retrospect and prospect. *Evaluation & the Health Professions, 18*(4), 349–369.

Loomis, M. E. (1985). Emerging content in nursing: an analysis of dissertation abstracts and titles: 1976–1982. *Nursing Research, 34*(2), 113–119.

McCormick, K. A. (1994). Preface. In K. A. McCormick, S. R. Moore, & R. A. Siegel (Eds.), *Clinical practice guideline development: Methodology perspectives* (AHCPR Pub. No. 95-0009, p. vii). Washington, DC: U.S. Department of Health and Human Services.

Mulrow, C. D. (1987). The medical review article: State of the science. *Annals of Internal Medicine, 106,* 485–488.

Mulrow C. D., & Oxman, A. D. (Eds.) (1994). Cochrane collaboration handbook [updated September 1997]. In The Cochrane Library [database on disk and CDROM]. The Cochrane Collaboration, Issue 4. Oxford: Update Software.

NHS Centre for Reviews and Dissemination. (1996). *Undertaking systematic reviews of research on effectiveness. CRD Guidelines.* York, England: NHS Center for Reviews and Dissemination.

National Institute of Nursing Research (NINR). (1993). *National nursing research agenda: Setting nursing research priorities.* Bethesda, MD: National Institutes of Health.

Olson, R. K., Heater, B. S., & Becker, A. M. (1990). A meta-analysis of the effects of nursing interventions on children and parents. *MCN: American Journal of Maternal–Child Nursing, 15*(2), 104–108.

Rice, R. R., & Richlin, L. (1993). Broadening the concept of scholarship in the professions. In L. Curry & J. F. Wergin (Eds.), *Educating profession-·als: Responding to new expectations for competence and accountability.* San Francisco: Jossey-Bass.

Sackett, D. L., Rosenberg, W. M. C., Gray, J. A. M., Haynes, R. B., & Richardson, W. S. (1996). Evidence based medicine: What it is and what it isn't. *British Medical Journal, 312*(7023), 71–72. (Available: http://cebm.jr2.ox.ac.uk/ebmisisnt.html#coredef.)

Shadish, W. R., Cook, T. D., & Leviton, L. C. (1991). *Foundations of program evaluation: Theories of practice.* Newbury Park, CA: Sage.

Sigma Theta Tau International (STTI). (1993). Manuscript guidelines for the *Online Journal of Knowledge Synthesis.* (Available: http://stti-web.iupui.edu/.)

Sigma Theta Tau International (STTI). (1998). Sigma Theta Tau International homepage. (Available: WWW.STTI-Web.IUPUI.EDU.)

Stetler, C. (1985). Research utilization: Defining the concept. *Image, 17*(2), 40–44.

Stevens, K. R. (1994, June). *The state of nursing science.* Presentation to American Nurses Association, San Antonio, TX.

Stevens, K. R. (1997, October 23). *Knowledge for clinical practice.* Presentation to Sigma Theta Tau Kappa Epsilon Chapter-at-Large, Grand Rapids, MI.

Stufflebeam, D. L., & Shinkfield, A. J. (1985). *Systematic evaluation.* Boston: Kluwer-Nijhoff.

Stufflebeam, D. L., & Webster, W. J. (1994). An analysis of alternative approaches to evaluation. In J. S. Stark & A. Thomas (Eds.), *Assessment and program evaluation.* Needham Heights, MA: Simon & Schuster.

Swanson, E. A., McCloskey, J. C., & Bodensteiner, A. (1991). Publishing opportunities for nurses: A comparison of 92 U.S. journals. *Image, 23*(1), p. 33–38.

Tanner, C. A., & Lindeman, C. A. (1987). Research in nursing education: Assumptions and priorities. *Journal of Nursing Education, 26*(2), 50–59.

Titler, M. G., Kleiber, C., Steelman, V., Goode, C., Rakel, B., Barry-Walker, J., Small, S., & Buckwalter, K. (1994). Infusing research into practice to promote quality care. *Nursing Research, 43,* 307–313.

Walker, L. (1982, May 23–25). *The present state of nursing research.* Presented at the Mabel Wandelt Research Day, Austin, TX.

Werley, H., Devine, E., Zorn, C., Ryan, P., & Westra, B. (1991). The nursing minimum data set: Abstraction tool for standardized, comparable, essential data. *American Journal of Public Health, 8*(4), 421–426.

Werley, H., & Lang, N. (1988). *Identification of the nursing minimum data set.* New York: Springer.

White, S. J. (1997). Evidence-based practice and nursing: The new panacea? *British Journal of Nursing, 6*(3), 175–178.

Zielstorff, R. D., Jette, A. M., & Barnett, G. O. (1990). Issues in designing an automated record system for clinical care and research. *Advances in Nursing Science, 13*(2), 75–88.

Chapter 2

Mentorship in Nursing Education

ROBERTA K. OLSON, PHD, RN
CONNIE VANCE, EDD, RN, FAAN

INTRODUCTION AND BACKGROUND

Mentorship in nursing education is an important element of professional and self-development that can lead to professional success and personal satisfaction. Research studies and anecdotal reports validate that having a mentor, or multiple mentors, enhances career development. The value of mentoring for professional socialization and scholarly productivity has been recognized by persons in every stage of their career. The challenge to nursing professionals is to create mentoring opportunities, including formalized mentor programs, for all levels of nursing students, for nurse educators, and for academic administrators, so that commitment to and leadership for the profession and scholarship are ensured.

Definition

According to Vance and Olson (1998),

> The mentor connection is a developmental, empowering, nurturing relationship extending over time in which mutual sharing, learning, and growth occur in an atmosphere of respect, collegiality, and affirmation. A mentor is someone who serves as a career role model and who advises, guides, and inspires another person, i.e., the protégé, during an extended period of time. Both mentor and protégé are developing and learning in the process. Therefore, a mentor can be a high-level professional or a peer-colleague. Appropriately, both mentoring partners should share an emotional investment and commitment to mutual development. From this perspective, it will be noted that mentoring is always relational, developmental, and longitudinal. It can also be complex, elusive, and difficult to quantify (pp. 4–5).

Historical Background

The word *mentor* is credited to Homer, in whose odyssey Mentor is the trusted friend of Odysseus left in charge of the household and his son during Odysseus's absence. Historically, a mentor was a wise guide and protector, possessing androgynous characteristics, who was also an ally, friend, supporter, and gift-giver. In the spiritual tradition of Taoism in ancient China, the secrets of legendary leaders, kings, and rulers were also contained in the principles of mentoring. These were based on insights into human nature, leadership succession, teaching and learning, and giving and receiving wisdom in all relationships (Huang & Lynch, 1995). Historically, especially in the corporate setting, mentoring has occurred between men, for example, the senior-to-junior relationship (Collins & Scott, 1978; Roche, 1979). Mentoring has been expected and systematically conducted between men. Today we see a rise of peer mentoring and, with women, a system of mentors at different points in the career trajectory. Women in female-dominant fields such as nursing, education, and social work are discovering the value of mentor relationships and are implementing different approaches, such as peer mentorships, that are suited for their developmental needs (Vance & Olson, 1998).

Many nursing leaders from Nightingale to contemporary leaders have experienced the benefits of having mentors (Fields, 1991; Schorr & Zimmerman, 1988). The first systematic investigation of mentor relationships among nursing leaders in the United States concluded that mentorship is present among identified nursing leaders, most likely contributing to the succession of leadership in the profession (Vance, 1977). These leaders diverged from the traditional model of mentoring; multiple mentors, in addition to the one all-encompassing mentor, were present and provided a wide variety of mentoring assistance. Peer colleagues and work supervisors were also especially important to nursing leaders, with the majority of their mentors being women. An early report of expert clinicians who mentored novice nurses found that each person in these developmental relationships experienced work satisfaction and that quality patient care was enhanced (Atwood, 1979).

Theoretical Foundation

Mentoring is a unique type of developmental relationship. Erikson's stage of generativity model (1963, 1968) is one developmental model that supports reaching out to others for guidance and nurturance. Inherent in generativity is the acceptance of responsibility for passing on wisdom to the next generation. As with mentoring, this developmental assistance provides a mutually enriching experience for the helper and the recipient.

Another theoretical foundation for mentoring is the social learning theory of Bandura (1977), which is based on imitation of modeling behavior of another person versus trial-and-error learning. The individual acquires a larger, better integrated behavior pattern more effectively and efficiently through modeling. Imitation of modeling behaviors is an inherent part of the mentor process throughout various stages of self-development and professional growth. The developmental stages of men and their mentoring relationship were described as "one of the most complex, and developmentally important [relationships], a man can have in early adulthood" (Levinson, Darrow, Klein, Levinson, & McKee, 1979, p. 97). In a later study, Levinson (1996) described mentor relationships for women: Women experience similar, but slightly different, stages of adult development in "life circumstances, in life course, in ways of going through each developmental period" (Levinson, 1996, p. 36). It is clear that women confront the developmental tasks of each stage with unique experiences, resources, and constraints.

O V E R V I E W

This chapter presents a review of the literature on mentorship in nursing education including undergraduate students, novice nurses, graduate students, nurse educators, and academic administrators. Three previous literature reviews summarize the research related to mentor relationships in nursing through 1988: Jowers and Herr (1990), Vance and Olson (1991), and Olson and Vance (1993). This chapter describes the research studies, opinion pieces, and related theoretical perspectives on mentor relationships that have been published since 1988, except for master's and doctoral dissertation research studies that are not as widely available and were published prior to 1988.

The scope of the literature reviewed included the electronic Cumulative Index to Nursing and Allied Health Literature (CINAHL), referral of articles from colleagues and personal article files from the past 15 years that are updated monthly through a continuous university library literature search on mentoring in nursing. A total of 67 articles were reviewed; 34 were excluded because they were cited in previous annual reviews, they were not relevant to mentoring in nursing education as research, or they were opinion pieces. A total of 33 research studies are cited. The chapter is divided into five sections: undergraduate nursing ($N = 8$), novice nurse/role transition to entry-level position ($N = 8$), graduate nursing (master's students, $N = 2$, and doctoral students, $N = 1$), nurse educator ($N = 7$), and academic administrator ($N = 7$). The five sections reflect specific skill application or guidance and formal programs for role preparation through mentoring. The research methodologies in each study discussed the design, valid and reliable instrumentation, and statistical findings. The research methodology in each study were judged by the authors of this chapter to be sound. The numbers of subjects in the studies ranged from 6 to 477.

RESEARCH RELATED TO MENTORING WITH UNDERGRADUATE NURSING STUDENTS

Undergraduate students have reported that mentoring experiences with teachers and clinical nurses improved their communication, technical, and organizational skills and facilitated transition into entry-level positions at graduation (Alvarez & Abriam-Yago, 1993; Atkins & Williams, 1995; Baldwin & Wold, 1993; Cahill & Kelly, 1989; Daly & Jones 1988; Larson, Hill, & Haller, 1993; Ramsey, Thompson, & Brathwaite, 1994; Turton & Herriot, 1989). The National Student Nurses Association (NSNA) adopted a resolution at its April 1996 convention supporting he promotion, awareness, and development of mentorship programs in schools and nursing organizations (NSNA, 1996). Early mentoring experiences for students can occur with faculty and staff nurses and with senior students serving as peer mentors.

The following four research reports reflect specific skill application by undergraduate students. In one report, selected senior students, through an independent study course, supervised sophomore students in an on-campus learning laboratory. These experiences reinforced the senior students' knowledge of the skills and facilitated implementation of teaching–learning principles (Daly & Jones, 1988). Staff nurse involvement with students in their psychiatric nursing clinical practicum was described by Turton and Herriot (1989). Each registered nurse (RN) served as a mentor in helping students learn the finer points of nursing interventions with psychiatric patients, which resulted in excellent recruitment and retention of entry-level nurses. A similar experience was related by Atkins and Williams (1995) in their description of the challenges for staff nurses who serve as mentors for students. The staff nurse mentors needed formal preparation in several areas: (a) understanding adult learning principles, (b) balancing the tension created by working intensively with another person, (c) understanding conflict resolution principles, (d) acknowledging the personal and professional development of mentors, (e) intensity of time involved, (f) maintaining a high level of commitment, and (g) gaining support from others in implementing the role of mentor, including peers, managers, and the nursing faculty. Despite these challenges, the majority of staff nurses felt rewarded by the satisfaction of helping future colleagues. Larson et al. (1993) described a clinical experience with RNs working with undergraduate students on research applications. The RNs identified a nursing practice on the patient unit of immediate concern and relevance to their clinical work, and the three to four students on the "research team" individually searched the literature, shared their results with the team, and wrote a report of their combined findings with recommendations. Four of the 22 projects resulted in changes in nursing practice.

The following four studies describe planned or formal mentor programs for undergraduate students (protégés). Junior students were linked with alumni "in the field" in a planned mentor program described by Cahill and Kelly (1989), the purpose of which was to provide reality and support for the students from experienced professionals. Program outcomes for the protégés included increased self-confidence, an opportunity to experience the work world prior to graduation, and transition into their first position as new graduate nurses. For the alumni mentors, the outcomes were enhancement of self-worth and their own professional development as well as an increased awareness of the needs of younger nurses and coworkers.

Completion of and satisfaction with the nursing program were the outcomes found by Baldwin and Wold (1993) in their pilot study with students from disadvantaged backgrounds. Mentor–protégé relationships were set up to provide disadvantaged students with faculty (mentor) support during the undergraduate program. The four mentored and four nonmentored students were asked to complete the researcher-developed level of satisfaction questionnaire. The four mentored students and two of the nonmentored students completed the questionnaire, and results indicated that these six students were equally satisfied with the nursing program. The four who were mentored cited many benefits from the mentor relationship, including support from the mentor, responses to specific problems, advice on course progression, and encouragement for future efforts. These students had frequent interaction with faculty during their academic program. Astin (1990) supported the finding that frequent interaction with faculty led to a higher level of satisfaction and personal and professional growth.

Alvarez and Abriam-Yago (1993) developed a program to improve the retention of ethnic students enrolled in one associate degree–nursing (ADN) and one bachelor of science–nursing (BSN) program in California. Goals established for the program included emotional support; a sense of the reality of becoming a nurse; basic skills in studying, writing, and speaking; and a pride in their diverse heritage, which is needed in health care providers. The RN mentors were recruited to facilitate this relationship, and the students were invited to apply. There were 46 student/RN pairs the first year and 22 the second year. The retention rate from the first year of the program was 44 graduates, or 96%. In another study, nursing professionals in the Queens County Black Nurses Association (QCBNA) evaluated their professional commitment for mentoring students of color in local baccalaureate nursing programs (Ramsey et al., 1994). The QCBNA mentors believed that nontraditional students over the age of 25 particularly needed the benefits of a mentor to grow beyond inherent prejudicial assumptions in the educational system. Ten of the QCBNA professional nurses worked with the deans of two colleges of nursing to identify 10 nursing students who met the objectives for the mentor program. The purpose of the project was to provide nurturance and support to facilitate successful completion of the baccalaureate program. At the time of their report, of the original 10 students, two had successfully completed the program and passed the National Council Licensure Examinations–Registered Nurse (NCLEX–RN); one did not meet academic requirements and was assisted by her mentor to change career direction, and the remaining seven were progressing satisfactorily. The volunteer mentors in this program established a contract of expectations with each protégé, and provided assistance with time management, development of good study habits, and strategies for stress reduction and test anxiety. In addition, the mentors encouraged the students to initiate early and frequent communication with the faculty. Because of its success, the program was expanded in the second year.

In these studies, undergraduate students who were mentored reportedly gained self-assurance and self-confidence and felt cared about as they progressed toward their professional and educational goals. Their mentors served as important role models and assisted in career planning. Reciprocal benefits of mentoring are illustrated in these studies, as the mentors believed that their teaching skills had been refined and that their own learning was stimulated through mentor relationships with students. Professional nurses who engaged in mentor partnerships with students found that their own personal and professional development was strengthened (see Table 2–1).

PROFESSIONAL ROLE TRANSITION OF THE NOVICE NURSE

The literature supports the importance of the first job in an individual's chosen profession. Mentoring of new graduates increases their self-assurance and confidence in skill performance. Clearly, interventions designed to socialize the new graduate nurse into the profession also benefit the employing organization through decreased orientation costs and time for recruitment and reorientation.

TABLE 2–1.
Undergraduate Students

Author/ Date	Purpose	Sample	Method	Findings
Alvarez & Abriam-Yago (1993)	Improve retention of ethnic students enrolled in both nursing programs—the ADN program at a community college and a BSN program at a state university. Goals established for the mentors: (1) provide emotional support to protégés, (2) assist protégés in working with faculty members, and (3) assist protégés in making the transition from student to RN. Goals established for the protégés: (1) improve performance in their nursing programs, and (2) recognize the value of their biculturalism in preparing them to meet the health care needs of a culturally diverse community.	Year 1: 46 undergraduate student protégés and 46 professional nurse mentors. Year 2: 22 protégés and mentors.	The program had five phases: recruitment of students and mentors, mentor training, matching protégés and mentors, mentor–protégé relationship, and evaluation. *Recruitment.* Students were enrolled in the ADN and the BSN programs. Mentors were professional nurses from hospitals and agencies in the community with ethnically diverse backgrounds. *Training.* Mentors received basic skills such as note-taking, preparing for and taking an exam, and time management. The second workshop centered on problem-solving strategies. Students received individual, informal orientation to the program the first year. The second year, the students received a more formal orientation to the process. *Matching the protégés and mentors.* The program staff assigned the matches using the information on the protégé's application and meeting with the mentors and protégés at the training or orientation sessions. The mentor–protégé dyad arranged the first meeting, discussed the expectations, signed a contract, and set up a time for the next meeting. *Mentor–protégé relationship.* The mentor–protégé dyad met once each month and had telephone contact every 2 weeks. Many became close friends. *Evaluation.* Extensive evaluation data were gathered on a written form and reported in the article.	The mentors reported enhancing their communication skills, serving as a support person and adviser, and discussing problem solving on a variety of topics of concern to the protégé. The protégé reported feeling supported; having someone to help with problems, gaining skills in leadership, communication with instructors, and networking strategies; gaining insight about nursing practice; and enhancing self-esteem. Ethnic minority student retention was 96% (44 of the 46) from the first year of the program. Mentor support was found to be essential.

TABLE 2–1.
Undergraduate Students (Continued)

Author/ Date	Purpose	Sample	Method	Findings
Atkins & Williams (1995)	Explore and analyze RNs' experiences in mentoring undergraduate students.	12 RN mentors of students.	Semistructured interviews, qualitative data analysis.	Mentoring is a complex and skilled activity: • Mentoring facilitates student learning. • Conflicts can occur between mentor and student. • Preparation for the role and support of the mentor are essential.
Baldwin & Wold (1993)	Determine if disadvantaged students achieve positive outcomes when engaged in frequent mentor–protégé interactions.	6 students, 4 mentored and 2 nonmentored, from disadvantaged backgrounds.	Research-developed, 10-item, Likert-type Level of Satisfaction Questionnaire, reviewed by 5 faculty members. A Cronbach coefficient alpha of .92 was determined. Qualitative questions including experiences that were beneficial or nonbeneficial.	Mentored students held higher expectations for their faculty; they had lower mean scores for attitude of faculty, quality of teaching, and challenge offered by the program.
Cahill & Kelly (1989)	Describe how a mentor program was planned for undergraduate students being matched with alumnae for "real" world experiences. Criteria were outlined for selection of students, alumnae mentors, and steps in setting up the experience. *Note.* These guidelines and assumptions about a planned mentoring program for undergraduate students have been cited in several subsequent publications on planned mentor programs.	A small pilot program was completed. No sample numbers were given.	Description of a planned mentor program for students (protégés) and alumnae (mentors). Criteria for the mentor and protégé selection were identified. Protégé: Undergraduate junior, 3.0 GPA, interested in particular clinical area, voluntary for 1 year, readiness as determined through personal interview. Mentor: 5–10 years nursing experience; in particular clinical area that matched with protégé interest; reference from employer regarding success in career; commitment to participate for 1 year; geographic proximity to protégé; willingness and enthusiasm as determined through personal interview.	Assumptions for protégés and mentors were provided from this study: *Protégés.* (a) students felt more confident; personal and professional identity was expanded; (b) networking was modeled; contacts led to positions following graduation; (c) students gained opportunity to experience "work world" (expanded contacts within community; gained a mentor/friend; gained insight into balancing work/family roles).

TABLE 2–1.
Undergraduate Students (Continued)

Author/ Date	Purpose	Sample	Method	Findings
Cahill & Kelly (1989) (*continued*)				*Mentors.* (a) self-worth increased when sharing knowledge with protégés; (b) had time to reflect on their careers; (c) were able to actualize Erickson's developmental phase of generativity; and (d) increased awareness of younger person's needs and desire to provide mentoring.
Daly & Jones (1988)	Through an independent study, a senior student developed three laboratory experiences for sophomore students. The senior student learned from her faculty–mentor; and served as a mentor–teacher for the sophomore students in facilitating learning in the three laboratory experiences.	8 sophomore students.	Senior student designed objectives and laboratory guidelines, set up learning stations, and provided demonstrations, guidance, and feedback to the sophomore students. The senior opened the lab for more practice hours and completed the mastery check-off of the sophomore students with the mentor faculty.	*Faculty–mentor.* learned from the senior student that (a) more one-to-one time was needed with sophomores, and (b) longer hours in the lab were needed to provide more practice opportunities for students. *Senior student protégé.* (a) learned more about nursing; (b) tailored activities to meet sophomore needs as identified by the senior; (c) learned that laboratory guidelines helped the sophomore students become better organized; and (d) learned that extra lab hours helped the sophomores become more confident and less anxious.

TABLE 2–1.
Undergraduate Students (Continued)

Author/ Date	Purpose	Sample	Method	Findings
Larson, Hill, & Haller (1993)	Prepare baccalaureate nursing graduates to apply research to clinical situations. Provide staff nurses with research findings to validate the research base for specific clinical practices and/or procedures within the educational and practice settings.	22 mentor staff nurses and 110 students (1 mentor and 3–4 students/ team).	Undergraduate students were teamed with staff nurses to use research to evaluate nursing practice at the hospital and, if indicated, recommend changes: (a) faculty assigned 3–4 students for one mentor staff nurse; (b) students contacted mentor staff nurse and set up meeting; (c) staff nurse presented one or more topics of immediate concern and relevance to their clinical work; group consensus was reached about the topic to be studied; each student observed the practice once, then independently did a literature review on the selected topic; (d) students each wrote a critique of pertinent research literature; a final report was written from the combined literature reviews with the guidelines of the staff nurse and faculty; and (e) final report and recommendations were presented in class and graded by the faculty.	*Protégés.* Viewed the application of research to clinical situations as very beneficial. The difficulty was scheduling meetings with a variety of class and work schedules. *Mentors.* Learned along with the students about applying research findings to change clinical practice. Four of the 22 projects resulted in changes in practice.

TABLE 2–1.
Undergraduate Students (Continued)

Author/ Date	Purpose	Sample	Method	Findings
Ramsey, Thompson, & Brathwaite (1994)	Identify at-risk students and facilitate retention and success in two baccalaureate nursing programs in the inner city (New York).	10 students and 10 QCBNA members. The ethnic minority students were having difficulty passing the NCLEX–RN. The mentors were members of the QCBNA.	The protégé students and mentor QCBNA members discussed the objectives of program retention and success on the NCLEX–RN. A contact was designed that delineated the responsibilities of both parties.	Two problems were identified: (a) the reluctance of some protégés to call their mentor or return their mentor's calls; and (b) the failure of several protégés to share major problems with their mentors. Several common needs were identified for the protégés: (a) assistance with time management, development of study habits, and strategies for reduction of stress and test anxiety; and (b) encouragement for protégés to initiate early and frequent communication with faculty. At the completion of the first year of the project, • 2 of the 10 successfully completed their NCLEX–RN examination. • 1 student left the program for failure to meet academic standards. • 7 students were progressing satisfactorily.

TABLE 2–1.
Undergraduate Students (Continued)

Author/Date	Purpose	Sample	Method	Findings
Turton & Herriot (1989)	Description of staff nurses in Birmingham, England, who worked on a psychiatric nursing unit and their mentoring experiences with nursing students. The syllabus covered all major specialities: acute, rehabilitation, community, and services for the elderly mentally ill.	3 students and 3 RN mentors.	The students were assigned to this integrated acute-admission mental health ward for a part-time 4-week rotation, then a 12-week full-time rotation with the RN mentors. The students had previously completed 8 months of training in general skills and nursing knowledge. A learning contract contained details that reflected expectations in a course syllabus and guided the teaching–learning process. The mentors attended a continuing education course on guiding and contracting to provide caring support and direction for the protégés.	There was a high level of commitment of the RN mentors to help the students become fully qualified as licensed nurses. Close liaison with the school of nursing was established. The students benefitted from a close relationship with the RN mentor to learn the clinical skills related to mental health nursing.

ADN = associate degree–nursing
BSN = bachelor of science degree–nursing
RN = registered nurse
QCBNA = Queens County Black Nurses Association
NCLEX-RN = National Council Licensure Examinations–Registered Nurse

Mentor programs can clearly facilitate the retention of new graduates (Andersen, 1989; Bellinger & McCloskey, 1992; Butts & Witmer, 1992; Carey & Campbell, 1994; Dufault, 1990; Martin, Tolleson, Lakey, & Moeller, 1995; Nayak, 1991; Schwerin, Gaster, Krolikowski, & Sherman-Justice, 1994).

Programs that facilitate work experience, along with clinical experience as a nursing student, enable the student to move smoothly into an entry-level staff position upon graduation. The Veterans Affairs Learning Opportunities Residency (VALOR) program with Veterans Administration Hospitals, in place since 1990, is one example (Martin et al., 1995). The student is paid as a nurse technician for 900 hours during the summer and two semesters prior to graduation. A project patterned after the VALOR program is in process with 10 baccalaureate students from Augustana College (Sioux Falls, SD) and South Dakota State University (Brookings, SD) with Sioux Valley Hospital, McKennan Hospital, and the Veteran's Administration Hospital (Sioux Falls, SD). The goal of this project is to provide these 10 individuals with a smooth transition into an entry-level staff position.

Andersen (1989) described development of the role of the nurse advocate to improve retention of new graduates, decrease attrition (turnover) of staff, and decrease recruitment costs. The seasoned RN nurse advocate worked closely with 30 new graduates and their preceptors with daily rounds, individual meetings, and focused activities to increase socialization and integration into the hospital environment. After 1 year, 29 of the new nurses were still employed; reduction of turnover and orientation reduced expenditures from $150,000 to $19,000 for the following year. Schwerin et al. (1994) had similar results with mentors and new nurses; in a carefully planned mentor program, attrition and orientation costs were significantly cut. Nayak (1991) described a similar study by collecting data about the work experiences of new graduates so that retention strategies could be developed. Nayak recommended that clinical experiences be designed so that the new nurse's skill level could continually be expanded with support from an expert nurse. "Debriefing" opportunities were needed so the new graduate had an opportunity to discuss difficulties, feel supported, learn new skills, and move forward with renewed confidence. The staff recognized that sensitivity to the needs of the new nurses, particularly during their first year of employment, meant the difference between retention of satisfied, long-term employees and rapid turnover. Bellinger and McCloskey (1992) reported findings similar to those of Nayak, that mentor RNs for the new nurses facilitated earlier social integration and a higher level of professionalism and satisfaction.

Dufault (1990) and Butts and Witmer (1992) examined aspects of role mastery of new graduates. Dufault examined role mastery of new graduates as measured by Schwerian's Six-Dimensional Scale of Nursing Performance (1978) at the time of appointment and after 3 months in the position. The total score decreased over the 3 months for 25% of the new nurses. Dufault theorized that even though this indicated a loss of self-confidence in the new nurses, perhaps their perceptions of their role mastery were more accurate at 3 months, since their clinical competencies were tested during this time interval. The findings of the Dufault study were unclear when novice nurses' and seasoned nurses' total scores were compared. This may have been because the Six-Dimensional Scale was used with experienced preceptors and head nurses, even though it was designed for novice nurses. Butts and Witmer (1992) examined the difference between expectations of the new nurse and the nurse manager. The average time was 90 days or 3 months until the nurse manager felt that the new nurse was "oriented" and could function more independently. The nurse managers identified nine areas that the new nurse exhibited when he or she was integrated (oriented) into the unit. When a seasoned staff nurse mentor was assigned to a new nurse, support was provided at critical times during the orientation phase of the job, turnover was reduced, and the staff were more professionally satisfied. Carey and Campbell (1994) did not find a strong relationship between need satisfaction and the presence of a mentor but did conclude that management strongly supported the development of supportive, interpersonal relationships among staff nurses, and when levels of satisfaction were improved with reward for outcomes, there was a lower level of staff turnover (see Table 2–2).

RESEARCH RELATED TO GRADUATE NURSING STUDENTS

Graduate students in both master's and doctoral programs report the importance of being cared about and receiving guidance, teaching, and encouragement from mentors. The majority of graduate students' mentors are faculty (Gjertsen, 1992; Hanson & Hilde, 1989; Hayes, 1994; Linc & Campbell, 1995).

Master's Students

Gjertsen (1992) studied 13 master's students in one practicum experience to determine the correlation between mentor relationships for the students and expansion of leadership skills. 46% of the students believed that a mentor relationship had developed through the support and encouragement they received in leadership skill application and career planning. The hypothesis was not supported, that is, that mentoring increased leadership effectiveness. The number in the study was perhaps too small for statistical significance. Linc and Campbell (1995) studied mentoring for master's students by linking nurse anesthetist students with faculty and anesthesiologists in ongoing research or developing proposals to investigate common nursing problems surrounding surgery and administration of anesthetics. One multidisciplinary group studied pain management and another examined the use of muscle relaxants for tonsillectomy and adenoidectomy and postoperative complications. The nurse anesthetist graduate students expressed satisfaction with the mentoring process in implementing principles of research in the clinical setting. The next phase of the project included second-year students in the mentoring role with first-year students and the multidisciplinary team. The students stated that this helped demystify the research process.

TABLE 2–2.
Novice Nurse Role Transition

Author/ Date	Purpose	Sample	Method	Findings
Andersen (1989)	Develop the role of the nurse advocate to improve retention of new graduates, decrease staff attrition (turnover), and decrease recruitment costs.	30 new graduates and 30 staff nurse preceptors.	A RN position as coordinator of nursing grants and special projects was created by deleting another coordinator position. Part of the responsibilities was a .3 budgeted position. This seasoned RN advocated for the 30 new graduate RNs with the following activities: (a) daily rounds on their units, (b) individual meetings, and (c) activities (i.e., guest relations workshops, role-playing, monitoring staffing patterns, and meetings with personnel involved with orientation). Each new RN was also assigned a preceptor.	One year after the 30 new RNs were employed, 29 were still on staff, decreasing expenditure for replacement of new graduates from $150,000 in 1987 to $19,000 in 1988. The nurse advocate role was highly satisfactory for the individual and served as a model for an experienced nurse in other settings.
Bellinger & McCloskey (1992)	Provide empirical data on the benefits of preceptorship programs for orientation of new RN graduates.	New RN graduates or seasoned RNs new to the unit—177 with preceptors and 98 without preceptors.	The McCloskey Reward/Job Satisfaction Scale (1974) was completed by the new graduates; data were gathered at three time periods—first 2 weeks on the job, and 6 and 12 months after employment. The scale has a test–retest coefficient of .79. The Cronbach alphas for each time period were .89, .89, and .90. Each subject's head nurse completed a performance evaluation on the new graduate and sent it directly to the researchers. Secondary data analysis was conducted on the Reward/Job Satisfaction Scale.	The preceptors were seen as a benefit for nurses with less experience and less education. The preceptors helped these nurses feel equally satisfied, socially integrated, and as professional as those with additional education. The researchers had hoped to find a higher level of satisfaction, social integration, and professionalism with less turnover and better performance with preceptorship programs.

TABLE 2-2.
Novice Nurse Role Transition (Continued)

Author/ Date	Purpose	Sample	Method	Findings
Butts & Witmer (1992)	Describe the distance between the nurse manager's expectations and the new RN graduates' abilities. Also, determine the relative importance attached to basic competencies, and the time frame in which the manager expects the new nurse to be independent in his or her practice.	35 nurse managers or assistant managers.	Critical incident technique was used to elicit activity requirements and ratings of urgency, importance, and independence of listed activities. Flanagan's (1954) technique of direct observation for specific behaviors was used. Experienced nurse managers identified nine competencies during Phase I indicative that new nurses were "oriented." The nurse managers identified what nurses do to show that they are proficient. These nine areas were (a) familiarity with nursing unit, (b) use of computer, (c) use of nursing process, (d) administration of medications without errors, (e) integration with coworkers into the setting, (f) administration of IV orders without errors, (g) appropriate use forms, (h) appropriate use of patient care equipment, and (i) patient care pre- and postop. During Phase II these nine areas were rated by the nurse managers according to importance and urgency in relation to time in which the task needed to be learned and whether the task performed at that time should be independent or required some supervision. The tasks parallel the content of the orientation program.	The nurse managers recognized that new graduates require at least 90 days or 3 months to feel independent and competent. During this transition time, a supportive mentor relationship with the manager and the staff nurse must occur. Also, the new graduate needs flexible time in the orientation schedule to learn the expectations of the job, develop a support group, identify his or her role, and discover a welcoming environment. When these basics are present, turnover is reduced and staff are professionally satisfied.

TABLE 2–2.
Novice Nurse Role Transition (Continued)

Author/ Date	Purpose	Sample	Method	Findings
Carey & Campbell (1994)	Determine if the use of preceptors, sponsors, or mentors for new RN staff would reduce turnover and cost of replacement.	143 staff nurses at 2 large hospitals.	Two questionnaires were distributed to the sample ($N = 230—20\%$ random selection of the total population of nurses): (a) a demographic form and the Moderating Beliefs and Work Results section of the Miller–Carey Role Inventory (1993) (acceptable levels of validity and reliability for these scales have been reported; Miller & Carey, 1993), and (b) the Fagan and Fagan Career Development Questionnaire (1983) with an additional section developed by the researchers.	The motivational needs of the nurses were being met at a high level as measured on the fulfillment and significance scales. There was not a strong relationship between need satisfaction and the presence of a mentor. Nurses left the organization because their professional needs for recognition, accomplishment, or sense of self-worth were not being met. The core of the reward outcome construct is support from members of management. *Conclusion:* When management strongly supports the development of supportive, interpersonal relationships, satisfaction with reward outcomes improves and turnover among staff nurses decreases. *Recommendation:* There is a need for a preceptor for the beginning professional, a mentor for the young professional, and a sponsor for the maturing professional.

TABLE 2–2.
Novice Nurse Role Transition (Continued)

Author/Date	Purpose	Sample	Method	Findings
Dufault (1990)	Explore the relative contribution of eight independent variables in explaining novices' (new nurse graduates) perceived variation in role mastery 3 months following their appointment.	75 novice nurses.	The eight independent variables were perceived level of role mastery of the novice upon entry, preceptor, head nurse, and nursing practice unit; previous work experience in nursing; job satisfaction on the unit; role socialization on the unit; and participation in bicultural training groups. The Schwerian Six-Dimensional Scale of Nursing Performance was administered to 96 novices, their 90 preceptors, and their 26 head nurses on the first day of orientation. The novice nurses were again tested at 3 months of employment (Schwerian, 1978). The Nursing Practice Group Role Mastery Assessment Scale, a revised version of Schwerian's instrument, was completed by nurse educators, who were familiar with the units, in rating the 26 nursing units' collective expertise, job satisfaction, and role socialization. All novice nurses, preceptors, and head nurses participated in the bicultural training.	The findings are unclear. The Six-Dimensional Scale of Nursing Performance was designed primarily to be used with experienced nurses, not with novice nurses who serve as preceptors and head nurses. 25% of the novice nurse scores for time of appointment and 3 months into employment reflected a decrease in their total score at 3 months. The decrease in score indicated a loss of self-confidence in the novice once the "honeymoon" phase was over. However, perhaps the perception of their role mastery was more accurate at 3 months following experiences in all six areas—leadership, critical care, teaching/collaboration, planning/evaluation, interpersonal relations and communication, and professional development. Bicultural training has been linked to decreased turnover, cost-effectiveness, and increased job satisfaction but was not addressed in the findings.

TABLE 2-2.
Novice Nurse Role Transition (Continued)

Author/ Date	Purpose	Sample	Method	Findings
Martin, Tolleson, Lakey, & Moeller (1995)	Describe the VALOR program. The purpose of the program is to have senior nursing students work at the VA hospital in a closely supervised RN role with a seasoned preceptor. The goal is for these students to move smoothly into staff nurse roles after graduation.	2 students within 1 year of graduation per participating VA hospital are accepted into the VALOR program.	Criteria for eligibility for selection include BSN students at the end of their junior year, minimum GPA of 3.0 on a 4.0 scale, and no grade lower than a B in any nursing course. The students are assigned to a preceptor. Intensive care units are frequently the selected clinical area, and the students' preferences are taken into account. Students receive additional information about services and have experiences throughout the hospital, plus attend classes and meetings such as critical care classes.	Facilities recruitment of high-level staff nurses, reduces orientation costs ($7,000 to $10,000 per student), decreases anxiety, and facilitates a seamless transition into the role of staff nurse. The students/new staff nurses indicate that their ability to process information, make clinical judgments, and perform nursing skills is greatly improved through the VALOR program.

TABLE 2-2.
Novice Nurse Role Transition (Continued)

Author/ Date	Purpose	Sample	Method	Findings
Nayak (1991)	Collect data about the work experiences of new graduates so that a retention strategy could be developed.	48 new graduates, divided into 4 groups.	Each of the four groups was assigned a nurse researcher who met with each participant. The 1-hour, individual, confidential meetings were conducted every 8 to 12 weeks with each new nurse. During the interviews, the new graduate was asked to describe a critical incident. The nurse researcher took field notes. The feelings and perceptions of support felt by the new graduate were recorded. The field notes were then coded for emerging themes.	Clinical critical incidents were cited 84% of the time. Sources of social support for 78% of the group were family and friends; the remaining 22% cited professional relationships as their social support. These 22% were identified as a high-risk group for being less able to cope with job-related stress when using professional relationships versus family and friends for social support. Resources used were the assigned preceptors during the first 4 months and peer support for the next 14 months. Positive work experiences were personal and professional accomplishments, contribution to the well-being of the patients, and verbal and physical support at work. A subgroup of new nurses (20%) was unable to find anything positive about the work experience; this group was the most at risk for attrition. The highest critical incident category for negative work experience (90%) was related to patient suffering and emergencies. These incidents created feelings of personal/professional inadequacy.

TABLE 2–2.
Novice Nurse Role Transition (Continued)

Author/ Date	Purpose	Sample	Method	Findings
Schwerin, Gaster, Krolikow-ski, & Sherman-Justice (1994)	Develop and implement a mentor program for role socialization of new nurse graduates.	56 new nurses in 1989, and 36 new nurses in 1992.	The mentors were selected on the basis of specific criteria that included familiarity with hospital policies and procedures, effective communication, expert clinical skills, ability to facilitate learning and provide feedback, and commitment to the mentor program and professional nursing. Orientation to the expectations of the role and follow-up meetings were required of the mentors. A mentor–new nurse (orientee) agreement was negotiated. Mentor responsibilities included assessing protégés' learning needs, ensuring learning opportunities, providing feedback, serving as role model and support resource, and promoting unit socialization. The protégé's responsibilities included identifying learning needs, seeking and completing the learning experience, providing feedback to the mentor, and using the mentor for professional and personal development.	The cost of the mentor workshops totaled $6,200 (this does not reflect the cost of replacing an experienced nurse with a new nurse). Prior to the mentorship program, the turnover rate was 19.5% on the medical–surgical units. In the 2 years after the mentorship program, turnover dropped to 11.6%. The 40% decrease reflected a savings to the hospital of $124,000/year in orientation costs alone.

BSN = bachelor of science–nursing
GPA = grade point average
MSN = master of science–nursing
RN = registered nurse
VALOR = Veterans Affairs Learning Opportunity Residency

The articles by Hanson and Hilde (1989) and Hayes (1994) describe methodologies for mentoring graduate students but are not research-based. Since the Nightingale era, it has been common for faculty to practice in a setting and directly mentor graduate students in clinical settings by serving as hands-on practitioners and including students in their own caseload. Hanson and Hilde (1989) described the richness of this ongoing practice in the community health setting, concluding that the clients are the "winners" in this mentorship arrangement. The importance of having nurse practitioners (NPs) mentor NP students was also described by Hayes (1994), in a study in which preceptors were assigned for a specific semester of clinical practicum. This preceptor relationship frequently developed into a longer term interaction that could be described as a mentor relationship.

Doctoral Students

Meleis (1992) discussed the scholarship growth that should occur during doctoral education, including the need for passionate scholarship that is driven by substance and sensitivity to cultural diversity and global collaboration. One of the suggested strategies to achieve this level of scholarship is through a series of mentors for the doctoral student, because one mentor may not be able to provide all that a doctoral student needs. In addition to developing scholarship, doctoral students also need to develop leadership skills. Several authors have written excellent, but non-research-based, articles on the role of mentoring for doctoral students (Davidhizar, 1988; Heinrich & Scherr, 1994; May, Meleis, & Winstead-Fry, 1982; Valverde, 1980; Waters, 1996). Only one evaluation study since 1988 on mentoring of doctoral students was located: Olson and Connelly (1995).

Olson and Connelly (1995) conducted an evaluation study on predoctoral students' experiences with application of research skills. A one-page proposal was prepared by each of the faculty (i.e., what they could offer) and the doctoral students (i.e., what they needed to strengthen their research skills). The students interviewed the faculty to learn more about a potential match. A committee external to the school of nursing selected pairs based on the proposals and rankings by the faculty and students. The researchers interviewed the four mentor–protégé dyads to determine if research productivity was increased through this planned experience. Interview data revealed that Yoder's (1990) model of mentoring was inherent in these relationships with the additional variables of socialization as a researcher and mutual sharing. Six themes emerged from the experiences as reported by the participants: productivity, work organization, mutual learning, problems encountered, beneficial research application skills, and innovative communication skills. The doctoral student protégés believed that their application of research went far beyond the usual experiences of a research assistant. They were involved in the following activities: grant writing, the National Research Service Award (NRSA) application process, management of a large grant, and mutual critique of presentations and manuscripts.

A peer-mentoring model supports the concept of framing teaching principles so that graduate students serve as "peers" in teaching each other, as described in an article on teaching strategies (Heinrich & Scherr, 1994). The purpose of the framework was to consult with peer graduate students in designing relevant learning experiences to meet objectives for student learning. The peer graduate group provided critique and feedback on the planning and presentation of the teaching episodes. The outcomes emphasized the value of peer mentoring for increased effectiveness in learning.

The importance of preparing ethnic minority nurse researchers was described by Waters (1996). Because the number of ethnic minority nurses, which is approximately 10% of the total nursing population, is low in relation to the general population, the nurse scientists who provide mentoring for ethnic minority nurses are frequently white and non-Hispanic. These individuals must be culturally competent in order to incorporate cultural sensitivity into research. Four factors critical to the survival and success of ethnic minority researchers are instructions in research expertise, affiliation with and mentoring by the research community, sustaining ethnic minority researchers' contributions in research, and increasing the number of ethnic minority researchers (Valverde, 1980; Waters, 1996).

Doctoral students need mentors to develop leadership skills, as emphasized in an opinion piece by Davidhizar (1988). Davidhizar indicated that a mentor is also a role model and preceptor, but a role model and preceptor are not necessarily mentors. The role of a mentor in developing leadership skills in doctoral students includes six characteristics: (a) forwardmindedness—goal-directed and envisioning the future for potential development of the protégé; (b) common interest—a significant match in research or other goals; (c) advice and strategies—on learning the leadership role and accomplishing other goals including growth of the protégé; (d) self-exposure—trust in the relationship that leads to self-disclosure, insights, requesting help, and problem solving; (e) affirmation—enhancement of self-esteem, recognition of protégé's potential, mutual admiration and respect for each other; and (f) development of protégés as mentors—so the protégé becomes the mentor in promoting the cycle of mentor relationships.

May et al. (1982) identified the importance of the development of the protégé as he or she becomes immersed in the process, learns new processes, and emerges with a new sense of direction, autonomy, identity, and goals. The protégé's perception of conflict and the solution were found to be crucial elements in the ability to develop with the mentor. Both enlargement of the protégé's perception and use of this specific process to develop and adjust to changed perceptions were identified by protégés as crucial to development within each phase. Protégés demonstrated a preference for their initial mentor. This cycle of self-development reflects Kegan's (1982) theory on maturing, which is the process of both differentiating self from others and integrating self with others. The balance throughout maturation is between self and other, and the continued tension of development comes from the need for inclusion and connectedness and the need for autonomy and independence (Johnsrud, 1991).

The importance of mentoring for scholarly productivity of doctoral students was described by May et al. (1982). While not a research report, the article discusses the essential role that a good mentor has in grooming novice scholars for their life's work, particularly in research. The need for trust and mutuality in the relationship is great, so that the novice scholar can "rehearse" with guidance to avoid "pitfalls" but at the same time can express innovative ideas. The mentor's scholarly work must be conceptually sound, premises explicit and well documented, and stated biases crystal clear. "Graduate school faculty have the awesome responsibility of providing a paradigm of the scholarly life, both by the quality of their performance and by the level of achievement they inspire and require" (May et al., 1982, p. 24).

It has been posited that doctoral educational standards must be high so that a community of scholars is educated to conduct research that leads to sound policy decisions, improves access to health care for diverse groups, and improves the science of nursing (Meleis, Hall, & Stevens, 1994). It is essential that diversity among doctoral students be embraced, and that collaborative mentorship be used to ensure a strong conceptual base for scholarship. Collaborative mentorship includes negotiated relations, mutual interactions, facilitative strategies, and empowerment (see Table 2–3).

RESEARCH RELATED TO MENTORING OF NURSING FACULTY

Nursing faculty need socialization into the academic role with regard to (a) balancing the workload of teaching, research, and service and (b) integrating the work of teacher, evaluator, and guide for students. Nurse educators frequently experience a paradigm shift from the role as expert clinician to novice educator. The new nurse educator can easily apply clinical skills from a knowledge base built over time, but it is another matter to oversee and facilitate learning and gently guide the clinical learning of a student.

Balancing the Role of Nurse Educator

The new nurse educator is in some ways caught in the middle—wanting to be recognized for what he or she knows so well and at the same time needing to have the same expertise in facilitating learning in others. A seasoned nurse educator—a mentor—can facilitate this transition. Several authors have reviewed the importance of mentoring in the career socialization of the neophyte nurse educator (Kavoosi, Elman, & Mauch, 1995; Megel, 1985; Pappas, 1988; Powell, 1990; Rollin, 1991; Taylor, 1992; Zimmerman & Yeaworth, 1986).

In an opinion piece, Megel (1985) underscored the importance of a mentor in socializing the novice faculty member. The mentor facilitated priority-setting so that the protégé avoided "overload." A similar theme was reflected throughout the interviews conducted by Pappas (1988) on role conflict. The 16 participants responded to questions about the role conflicts among teaching, service, and research. Effective coping strategies focused on

TABLE 2–3.
Graduate Nursing Students

Author/ Date	Purpose	Sample	Method	Findings
Master's students Giertson (1992)	Explore the relationship and correlation of mentor experiences and the expansion of leadership skills among MSN students in one university course.	12 master's students in nursing.	The Leadership Effectiveness and Adaptability Description (LEAD-Self) tool was used to collect data prior to and at the completion of the role practicum for the graduate course in the quasi-experimental study (Stogdill, 1963).	The hypothesis that leadership effectiveness would increase as a result of mentorship was not supported. The number in the study was perhaps too small for statistical significance.
Linc & Campbell (1995)	Describe the mentoring strategies used by faculty with nurse anesthesia students.	14 nurse anesthesia students who were divided into 3 groups for the research project.	Descriptive study of a multidisciplinary approach to nursing research, with the students working with the anesthesiologist and the nurse researcher. One group studied pain management in patients. One set of patients received thoracic and lumbar epidural infusions of low-dose local anesthetics; the second set of patients received narcotics for postoperative pain management. A second group designed a study of the use of a clinical mentor and the perceived anxiety level of students in the clinical setting. The study was not completed by these students during their research course. A third group developed a proposal to study the effects of the use of muscle relaxants for tonsillectomy and adenoidectomy in children and postoperative complications. The study received approval but was not completed during the course. One outcome was that the first-year students became interested in this project. They were mentored by the second-year students as they assisted in the project while the nurse researcher and anesthesiologist mentored the second-year students.	This multidisciplinary approach to mentoring the research process in nurse anesthesia students was deemed beneficial. The students learned to design and gain approval for proposals in the research class. The actual implementation and data analysis of the studies were not required for the course, but many studies were completed during the next semester for the thesis requirement.

TABLE 2–3.
Graduate Nursing Students (Continued)

Author/ Date	Purpose	Sample	Method	Findings
Doctoral students Olson & Connelly (1995)	Determine if research productivity was increased through planned experience when the doctoral student worked 20 hours/week with a faculty member.	4 mentors (faculty) and 4 protégés (doctoral students).	Descriptive qualitative study using semistructured interviews and a written questionnaire. The faculty and predoctoral students were matched on faculty expertise and the student's need for research application skills, determined from a 1-page proposal from the student and interviews with the faculty. Questions for the interview focused on the research activities, types of interactions, and specific behaviors of the faculty–student dyad that were helpful, or not helpful, during the 12-month fellowship period. The interviews were tape-recorded, and qualitative data analysis (Miles & Huberman, 1984) was used to determine if each case (faculty–student pair) fit the theoretical model of mentoring as presented by Yoder (1990). The written questionnaire responses were used to validate data provided in the interviews.	Based on Yoder's model, the data from these 4 pairs support the working hypothesis that these fellowship pairs represented mentor relationships. Each characteristic of mentoring in Yoder's model emerged from the interview data, plus 2 additions—socialization as a researcher and mutual sharing. The doctoral students were heavily involved in the research of their faculty mentor and with their own research application skills. The 4 pairs were involved in grant writing, a NRSA application process, management of a large grant, and mutual critique of presentations and manuscripts. They believed that the outcomes went beyond the usual experiences of a research assistant. 6 themes emerged from the data: productivity, work organization, mutual learning, problems encountered, beneficial research application skills, and innovative communication skills.

MSN = master of science–nursing
NRSA = National Research Service Award

personal prioritizing of cognitive and emotion-focused strategies that included being well-organized, setting goals, staying on track, and seeking a mentor relationship. The study by Pappas is not cited in Table 2–4 because it does not focus on mentoring but rather focuses on role conflict.

Powell (1990) and Rollin (1991) conducted similar studies that sought information on how female nursing faculty benefitted from a mentor relationship. In both studies, role socialization and development of professional skills were facilitated, and career direction and progression were better focused.

Taylor (1992) studied mentor relationships in female nurse academicians ($N = 477$). The participants responded to a self-administered questionnaire that contained a modified format of five mentor scales developed by Gilbert (1985). The participants reported that mentoring was relevant in academia as one means for enhancing job satisfaction, increasing commitment, and ultimately increasing scholarly productivity of nurse academicians.

In a descriptive study, Zimmerman and Yeaworth (1986) determined factors that influenced career success in nursing. Responses were obtained from 194 doctorally prepared female nurses who reported career success. Ranked as most important in facilitating career success were personal characteristics: knowledge, intelligence, and competence. Ranked second was educational preparation at the doctoral level, and ranked third was the presence of significant others—teachers, peer/colleagues, and supervisors who provided mentoring. Doctoral education provided credibility, prestige, and opportunities for positions that were new, were challenging, and offered greater financial reward. Encouragement, support, and advice from a mentor for a career move were cited as important in career success and satisfaction. Advice for novice nurses was to (a) obtain correct and sufficient education, (b) set goals and plan their careers, (c) know and believe in themselves, and (d) network and secure a mentor.

The relationship between senior nursing faculty who mentored junior faculty and support for faculty from academic administrators was reported by Kavoosi et al. (1995). The 80 academic administrators and 389 senior nursing faculty from National League for Nursing (NLN)–accredited master of science programs responded through two written questionnaires. The responses revealed that 25% did not mentor faculty, but 75% did report mentoring. The three top-ranked professional activities were teaching about the job, demonstrating trust, and sponsoring the faculty member. Reports of administrative formal support for mentoring were minimal, but senior faculty reported that mentoring junior faculty was a professional obligation, and they were rewarded for mentoring behaviors through informal processes.

Scholarship Productivity

Scholarship productivity for faculty was further described by Butler (1989), Megel, Langston, and Creswell (1988), Watson (1990), and Wocial (1995). A plan for development of research skills in a university setting was outlined by Watson (1990). The academic administrators offered seed money for pilot

TABLE 2–4.
Nurse Educator

Author/ Date	Purpose	Sample	Method	Findings
Butler (1989)	Study the relationship between mentoring for the academic role and scholarly productivity among nursing faculty.	305 doctorally prepared nurse faculty.	The researcher developed an instrument to quantify scholarly productivity and solicit data on mentor experiences. An *ex post facto* descriptive correlation procedure was used to examine the study variables. A questionnaire designed by the researcher was mailed to doctorally prepared female nursing faculty who were employed full-time at NLN-accredited schools of nursing with graduate programs.	Mentoring for the academic role occurred for 55.7% of the participants. Scholarship productivity was enhanced when the mentor relationships focused on the research activities of the academic role. Three characteristics of the mentor relationship influenced the level of scholarship productivity: length (more than 2 years); timing (when the relationship cut across two or more periods of career development); and types of support (sponsor on ideas and projects, intense relationship, friendship, and philosophical similarity with mentor). Scholarship productivity was not ensured with every mentor relationship.
Kavoosi, Elman, & Mauch (1995)	Investigate the relationship between senior nursing faculty mentoring activities and support for faculty mentoring provided by nursing program administrators.	80 administrators and 417 senior faculty.	This study was descriptive and correlational. Two surveys were used: the Administrative Data Questionnaire (ADQ) (Kavoosi, 1992), and the Alleman Mentoring Scales Questionnaire (AMSQ) (Alleman, 1987). The ADQ was tested for reliability; the AMSQ had been tested with good reliability. The top three mentoring activities reported by faculty were teaching about the job, demonstrating trust, and sponsoring the faculty member.	There was no statistical significance between administrative support for mentoring and the type and extent of mentoring activities reported by senior nursing faculty. A formal program for mentoring did not impact the amount of mentoring any more significantly than did conceptual or no support for mentoring. Senior faculty believed that mentoring junior faculty was an important part of their own professional identity.

TABLE 2–4.
Nurse Educator (Continued)

Author/ Date	Purpose	Sample	Method	Findings
Megel, Langston, & Creswell (1988)	Examine the scholarly productivity of 96 academic faculty researchers in 47 NLN-accredited schools/colleges of nursing.	96 doctorally prepared nurse researcher faculty.	A researcher-developed instrument, the Survey of Scholarly Productivity, was used to collect the data. The instrument had three sections: demographic data, research productivity, and factors that influence scientific research productivity. A conceptual model outlined the correlates of productivity, intervening variables, and measures of scholarly productivity.	The majority of participants were female, were doctorally prepared, and had been in their current institutions for 7+ years. Participants were divided into 4 groups according to the number of research articles published in the past 3 years: none, 1–4, 5–7, and 8–16. The average for all participants was 1 research article, 1 nonresearch article, and 1–2 conference papers presented each year. The pattern of variability indicated that there was a high level of activity after the doctorate and through tenure, with a sharp decline following tenure. The most highly productive participants: (a) were motivated by peer researchers outside their own institution and their own research team versus internal motivation; (b) tended to coauthor papers with their mentors in graduate school, spent less time in teaching and more in administrative work, and had access to word processing via the computer; and (c) enjoyed conducting research and writing articles.

TABLE 2–4.
Nurse Educator (Continued)

Author/Date	Purpose	Sample	Method	Findings
Powell (1990)	Assess the ways in which mentors have been used by female nursing faculty members with an earned doctorate in university settings, and describe the process and outcomes of mentorship for those who have experienced this process.	26 nursing graduate faculty in Research I and II schools.	Data were collected with a brief demographic questionnaire and open-ended questions in telephone interviews. Questions about the mentor relationship were explored.	Protégés reported that the mentor relationship contributed to academic role socialization and development of professional skills; this led to more focused career progression. The mentor relationships varied in length, from 4 to 33 years. All reported that over time the relationship became more collegial and a friendship developed. The level of intensity lessened the longer the relationship continued.
Rollin (1991)	Describe the prevalence, characteristics, perceptions, and feelings of nurse educators with respect to their mentor–protégé relationships.	31 nurse educators from one nursing school with bachelor's and master's programs.	The self-administered questionnaire by Spengler (1982) was used to gather quantitative and qualitative data.	It was found that 82.6% had at least one mentor. Less than 50% rated their mentor as very important to their career development. And 43% believed that mentoring by senior graduate faculty of junior faculty in undergraduate programs was important to foster growth in these faculty.

TABLE 2–4.
Nurse Educator (Continued)

Author/ Date	Purpose	Sample	Method	Findings
Taylor (1992)	Assess the frequency, characteristics, and importance of the mentor–protégé relationship among female nurse academicians.	477 female nurse academicians in public, NLN-accredited nursing programs in the southern United States.	This descriptive study consisted of a self-administered questionnaire packet of a demographic data sheet and a modified format of 5 mentor scales developed by Gilbert (1985) and Pierce (1983).	Helpful to the protégé were discussions of strategies to handle professional situations, observing the mentor in professional situations, and providing opportunities for participation in professional activities. Important characteristics of the mentor-protégé relationship included the mentor's willingness to value protégés as people, ability to provide professional advice when needed, and belief in the potential of the protégé. The protégé reported that important power and achievement characteristics were mastery of concepts and ideas and capacity to work hard. The personal qualities of the mentor that the protégés considered of great importance were integrity, professional values, and trustworthiness. The highest rated qualities of the protégé's achievement were gaining confidence, enjoying work, and resolving conflicts.

TABLE 2–4.
Nurse Educator (Continued)

Author/ Date	Purpose	Sample	Method	Findings
Zimmerman & Yeaworth (1986)	Examine educational preparation, personal characteristics, and significant others in career success of women in nursing.	194 doctorally prepared female nurses.	A random sample was selected from the 1,834 names in the Directory of Nurses with Doctoral Degrees (ANA, 1980). There were 282 names originally selected; of these, the adjusted sample was 236 with 194 returning the questionnaires, or a return rate of 82%. The investigator-developed Career Success Survey contained three selections: educational preparation, others who assisted and types of assistance provided, and self-assessment of personal characteristics. The questionnaire was mailed to the sample of 236.	Educational preparation was identified as giving the nurse more credibility and prestige, which opened up job opportunities and new challenges with greater financial rewards. Teachers, peer/ colleagues, and supervisors were the 3 top-ranked significant others who had an impact on career success. Types of assistance were encouragement, recognition of potential, confidence in the nurse, and help with career moves—identified as assistance from a "mentor." Self-assessment of personal characteristics revealed the four highest rankings as responsibility, knowledge, intelligence, and competence. Feelings of being successful were frequently related to salary.

ANA = American Nurses Association
NLN = National League for Nursing

studies and small projects and funds for research assistants and consultants; disseminated information about funding sources; and provided clerical support systems for submitting grant applications. Faculty members identified the category they preferred, and qualified for, in the research team. The team membership was lead researcher, researcher–teacher, or member. The team met to exchange ideas and set the research agenda during biweekly meetings, and faculty research skills were further cultivated during monthly seminars. Watson concluded that the doctoral graduate has excellent theory and some practical application but needs to link with a seasoned nurse researcher to maintain a research program.

Mentoring was the one variable that made the difference in scholarly productivity for faculty in a study of 305 participants by Butler (1989). Faculty responded to a questionnaire that explored the relationship between mentoring for the academic role and scholarly productivity. The three major influences of the mentor relationship, as described by the participants, were length of the mentorship, period of time when it occurred, and types of support provided by the mentor. The scores were higher when the mentorship took place over two or more years during doctoral study, or spanned two or more stages of career development, and when a variety of supportive functions were offered. Supportive functions included sponsorship of the protégés' ideas or projects that led to successful endeavors. An intense relationship, development of friendships, and philosophical similarity with the mentor were ranked as most significant for the protégé.

Megel et al. (1988) examined the scholarly productivity of 96 nurse faculty. The factors that contributed to a high level of productivity included (a) motivation by peers both outside their institution and on their own research team, (b) publications with faculty during graduate school, (c) less time in teaching and more in administration, and (d) enjoyment of conducting research and writing articles. A study conducted to determine factors that support and inhibit scholarly writing and publication included interviews with 59 women in academics from 13 colleges (Creamer, 1996). Their identified priorities were "(a) validation or confirmation of identity as a writer and scholar; (b) opportunities for development of skills in scholarly research, writing, and publication; (c) a culture of scholarship that provides socialization to the importance of scholarly research and writing, often through role models; and (d) a network of collegial relationships within and outside the institution, often through professional associations" (Creamer, 1996, p. 8). This nonnursing study concurs with the findings of Megel et al. (1988).

The essence of academic mentoring is that most faculty have developed a high level of clinical competence through experience and application of advanced skills in their graduate study. Learning the role of teacher, evaluator, and facilitator for students is enhanced with the help of a seasoned nurse educator mentor who can help shorten the learning time by coaching, role modeling, and providing feedback. The research program that the nurse educator needs to establish is supported with the help of a seasoned educator who has a research program in place. The nurse researcher who receives successful mentoring in the research process increases self-confidence and experiences greater success in funded ventures (Wocial, 1995). Wocial believes that a well-defined mentoring relationship is one strategy to nurture integrity and prevent scientific misconduct in research. Concentration of clinical practice, teaching, and research in one area with a primary focus, for example, pain management, reduces fragmentation for the novice nurse educator. A seasoned mentor can facilitate this focus (see Table 2–4).

RESEARCH RELATED TO MENTORING OF ACADEMIC ADMINISTRATORS

Academic administrators report the need for mentoring in the following areas: setting priorities, using consultants for new or difficult areas, and envisioning the "big picture." Academic administrators assume a broader level of accountability and responsibility and have greater access and authority over resources, so moving from a faculty role to that of academic administrator requires a broader perspective. Empirical and anecdotal studies have investigated the importance of mentoring career development and success of academic nurse-administrators (Gaspar, 1990; Laird, 1992; Lamborn, 1991; Larson, 1994; Princeton & Gaspar, 1991; Rawl, 1989; Rawl & Peterson, 1992; Redmond, 1991; Short, 1997a, 1997b).

Rawl (1989) examined variables that were relevant to career and leadership development in academic administrators. These variables included early life influences, academic preparation, mentoring relationships, supporting and constraining factors, and ways that the variables were relevant to the level of career development achieved. The participants' responses from 427 (71%) mail questionnaires revealed that mentoring did contribute significantly to their career development. However, in responses to the Scholarly Difficulty Index and the Work Commitment Index, participants indicated that highest degree and number of years as an academic administrator were factors more important in their career development (Rawl & Peterson, 1992).

The work satisfaction of nursing academic administrators was studied by Gaspar (1990). Telephone interviews with 32 subjects revealed that job satisfaction was enhanced when there was perceived influence on the organizational climate for development and change, control, facilitation of faculty growth and development, and lack of faculty conflict. Decreased job satisfaction themes were conflict, university constraints, lack of/need for control, organizational structure, and paperwork. Recommendations from the study included the need for doctoral-level preparation that included theory and application of social systems, organizational systems, management, and human behavior within organizations. Mentoring from administrative peers was also noted as important for job satisfaction (Princeton & Gaspar, 1991).

Redmond (1991) studied deans' perspectives on their lives, career relationships, and significant experiences that were important in assuming the role of dean. Themes that emerged from the data analysis included (a) patterns that strongly valued education and achievement, (b) supportive relationships with females for career guidance, and (c) early leadership experiences that led to enjoyment or a desire to be in charge. Lamborn (1991) examined factors that influenced job satisfaction and motivation of 595 deans and directors of schools of nursing. Mentoring was not identified as important in job satisfaction; rather, high job satisfaction resulted when there was a high level of motivation to do well in the position.

Laird (1992) studied the participants in the first Executive Development Series of the American Association of Colleges of Nursing (AACN). The major benefit of the series was development of collegial relationships that could serve in future networking, consultation, and problem solving. Other benefits identified were understanding the need for sufficient resources—staff, time, and budget—to perform well, and self-realization and confidence that they could perform in the role.

Larson (1994) examined career aspirations of academic middle managers (department heads and associate deans) to the role of dean or director. Responses from a mail questionnaire were received from 37 midlevel managers from 30 (of the 40 possible) schools of nursing in seven upper midwest states. Factors investigated included (a) satisfaction as measured by the Faculty Satisfaction Instrument (Johnson, 1979), (b) perceptions of powerlessness as measured by the Health Care Work Powerlessness Scale (revised) (Guilbert, 1979), and demographic characteristics. Larson found that a majority of the midlevel managers did not have career aspirations to a higher leadership level. The two major barriers for upward mobility in their careers were family responsibilities and lack of desire for more responsibility. The major barrier identified in the work environment was lack of support from the dean. Larson concluded that the dean holds the key for effective leadership development of faculty and managers through support, influence, and leadership in facilitating career advancement.

Short (1997a, 1997b) conducted a study with 324 deans and directors of AACN member schools to gain information on the perceived importance of various resources, participation in a mentor relationship, and various mentor functions. The major resources identified were excellent communication and interpersonal skills, creativity in thinking, ability to mobilize groups, and intellectual ability. Participants also indicated that one of the major influences for success was having multiple mentors who guided career development plus a broad background of experiences that assisted them in meeting the expectations of their roles.

These studies reveal the continuing need for a mentor relationship in learning the role of academic administrator. Educational preparation at the doctoral level in organizational behavior, knowledge of finance, and strategic planning is key to move from the narrower perspective of faculty or department head to that of academic administrator who is responsible for managing internal and external affairs for the college. An experienced mentor facilitates this career mobility and success. The AACN's semiannual Executive Development Series on the role of the academic administrator has been invaluable for prospective deans in gaining a perspective on the magnitude of the role, how to garner needed resources, and fiscal accountability (Booth, 1992) (see Table 2–5).

TABLE 2–5.
Academic Administrators

Author/ Date	Purpose	Sample	Method	Findings
Laird (1992)	Explore whether a professional development program could prepare nurses for the leadership role of dean. Survey participants of the AACN's first Executive Development Series to determine their perceptions of the program's influence on their professional development.	64 nursing faculty who were preparing for a deanship, 16 current deans, and 10 former deans.	A convenience sample of the 96 participants in the first Executive Development Series were mailed a questionnaire developed by the investigator. The questionnaire had fixed-alternate and open-ended questions.	83% of the prospective deans would consider a deanship if there were sufficient support staff, time for scholarship and research, and sufficient budget. The three top skills of a dean were formulating long-range goals, political savvy, and public speaking. The major benefit of the series was developing expert collegial relationships. A few respondents described the self-realization and self-confidence that occurred as a result of participating in this professional development opportunity. 23 of the 26 deans or former deans indicated that they initiated a mentor relationship with a prospective dean during this development series.

TABLE 2–5.
Academic Administrators (Continued)

Author/Date	Purpose	Sample	Method	Findings
Lamborn (1991)	Examine factors influencing job satisfaction of deans of nursing schools.	595 deans and directors of NLN-accredited bachelor's degree programs.	3 questionnaires were mailed to the participants. The first questionnaire collected demographic data; the second was the Motivation and Reward Scale, which measured motivation (Herrick, 1974); and the third was the Job Description Index (JDI), which measured components of job satisfaction (Smith, Kendall, & Hulin, 1969).	The demographic profile of deans of nursing is more homogeneous than previously reported. There is a strong correlation with high job satisfaction and a high level of motivation to do well. Job satisfaction resulted from positive outcomes from their efforts at facilitating needed change. Only half of the participating deans had any formal preparation for the role of dean. A number of responses indicated the high need for deans to be recognized and acknowledged by their peers—both professionally and for their academic ability. In keeping with expectancy theory, an overwhelming majority of the deans believed that, with effort, they could bring about an effective administration and meaningful change.

TABLE 2–5.
Academic Administrators (Continued)

Author/ Date	Purpose	Sample	Method	Findings
Princeton & Gaspar (1991)	Examine the role characteristics, responsibilities, and anticipated career patterns of first-line nurse administrators (department chairpersons, division directors, or coordinators) who were employed in university-based nursing programs throughout the United States.	56 first-line administrators.	An exploratory and descriptive survey was conducted with telephone interviews and mailed questionnaires. Four areas were explored: formal educational preparation; administrative competencies; coping strategies for conflicts, strains, and work overload; and anticipated career pattern.	33% had completed administrative courses in graduate school and had worked with administrative mentors. Two important competencies were having character and integrity. Setting priorities was the greatest strain, and work overload was dominant. 50% of the participants did not plan to continue in the administrative role because of the workload.
Redmond (1991)	Describe deans' perspectives on the life and career relationships and experiences that were significant to them in the assumption of the dean's position.	53 deans of nursing.	This study was a naturalistic design to discover developmental phenomena in deans' lives. Data were collected by survey, life history interviews, and a document search of curriculum vitae. Field notes were kept on the incoming data. Data were analyzed using Spradley's ethnographic analysis techniques, which consisted of domains, taxonomies, components, and themes.	The following themes were noted: (a) strong valuing patterns for education and achievement, (b) supportive relationships with females for career guidance, and (c) early leadership experiences that led to enjoyment or desire to be in charge. Conclusions: (a) frameworks such as Erickson, Levinson, Morgan, and Farber were useful, (b) people and relationships are important in career pathways, (c) early experiences in socialization and relationships facilitated leadership and positive ego development, and (d) strong values for achievement and education in early family and educational experiences and relationships were important.

TABLE 2–5.
Academic Administrators (Continued)

Author/ Date	Purpose	Sample	Method	Findings
Rawl & Peterson (1992)	Analyze the influence of mentoring on the level of career development of nursing education administrators. Other factors examined: early life influences, academic preparation, supporting factors, constraining factors, and career stages.	427 nursing education administrators from NLN-accredited schools.	An investigator-developed questionnaire was mailed to 600 randomly selected nursing educational administrators with a response rate of 71%. The 59-item questionnaire elicited information on career development, aspirations, mentoring experiences, and demographic data.	Mentoring contributed significantly to the level of career development. 9 other variables contributed to the achievement level of the administrator: highest degree earned, number of years since completion, number of years as an academic administrator, the scholarly difficulty index, the work commitment index, mentor relationships, number of months of nonemployment, number of children, and type of institution where highest degree was earned.

TABLE 2–5.
Academic Administrators (Continued)

Author/ Date	Purpose	Sample	Method	Findings
Short (1997a & b)	(1997a) To determine the perceived importance of various resources in the goal achievement of administrators of nursing schools. (1997b) Examine the current activities of influence for the deans, degree of participation in mentoring, and which mentoring functions were considered most important.	324 deans and directors of AACN member schools.	The questionnaire included the Profile of Influential Nurse Administrators and the 24-item Sources of Influence (Vance, 1977). These instruments were used to solicit data on the perceived importance of various characteristics and abilities that helped influential nurses achieve goals.	(1997a) The 5 top resources were identified as communication, interpersonal skills, creativity in thinking, ability to mobilize groups, and intellectual ability. Ranked lower, but perceived as important, were work or professional organization positions and mentoring. (1997b) A majority had entry-level bachelor's degrees and a doctorate. Only 27% reported a current mentor, but all had had mentors. Psychosocial function of a mentoring relationship was more important than career functions. Other highly influential activities were publications, presentations, serving as a consultant, and conducting research. Perceived influences for success were multiple mentors; various avenues of role preparation (including education); and scholarly, professional, and administrative expectations of the role.

AACN = American Association of Colleges of Nursing
NLN = National League for Nursing

IMPLICATIONS OF MENTOR RELATIONSHIPS IN NURSING EDUCATION

In every aspect of nursing education, from undergraduate nursing student experiences to the academic administrative role, mentor relationships have been identified as an essential component for personal growth and professional development. Informal mentoring includes peer mentoring along with the traditional expert-to-novice model. Informal or unplanned mentoring is guided by a mutual attraction between mentor and protégé; the mentor recognizes the potential in the protégé, or the protégé seeks a mentor who can provide developmental guidance. Planned or formal mentor programs are more deliberate, less dependent on mutual attraction, and beneficial for larger numbers of individuals. Planned mentoring with undergraduate and graduate students by peers, faculty, and professional nurses helps students apply knowledge and skills from the classroom to clinical practice. Planned organizational mentoring in colleges of nursing link new faculty with seasoned faculty to learn the role of educator and with researchers to learn the role of researcher/scholar. A community of scholars who emphasize caring, connectedness, and collaboration is essential in transmitting the norms and values of the academy to the next generation through mentoring (Johnsrud, 1991). Women bring affiliation, collaboration, and sharing to their work in academe, values that promote scholarly productivity that enable growth toward interdependence. Johnsrud contrasts this to the traditional one-to-one mentoring dyad that promotes accomplishment, competition, and scholarly isolation. She underscores the importance of a "community of scholars who are committed to the mutual growth and development of all of its participants" (Johnsrud, 1991, p. 16).

CONCLUSIONS

1. Mentoring phenomenon should be studied from a qualitative approach, as well as, from the current empirical methodology in order to more freely capture the rich character and complexity of the process.
2. There is a paucity of literature on planned (formal) and unplanned (informal) mentoring for graduate students. Specifically, no studies were located that describe the establishment of research programs following doctoral education through a formal mentoring process. Excellent opinion pieces are offered on the importance of scholarly caring in relation to increased productivity.
3. Scholarly productivity of nursing educators is reportedly enhanced with mentoring; however, both prospective and retrospective studies should be designed and implemented.
4. Phenomenological methods, using a case study approach with female academic leaders, will demonstrate how mentoring worked for them in a patriarchal culture. For example, how were barriers negotiated and obstacles turned into opportunities? (M. Barab, personal communication, June 23, 1997)
5. Research on collective and planned mentoring programs for students and faculty will illustrate the most useful ingredients in promoting professional success and personal satisfaction.

6. Replication of the mentoring studies cited, with increased sample sizes, should provide stronger evidence of the benefits and barriers of mentor relationships.
7. Instrument development will provide more valid and reliable measures of mentor relationship processes and outcomes.

Recommendations

Assuming responsibility for assisting future generations of practitioners, educators, and researchers through mentor relationships should be the norm in nursing, not the exception. Erikson (1963, 1968) emphasized "generativity" and the need to reach out to the next generation. Mentoring should not be an isolated phenomenon but should be integrated into every aspect of professional life for student through high-level leader. Scholarly productivity through teaching, research, and service activities is the tripartite mission of colleges and universities. Mentorship is a key process in facilitating scholarly productivity, clinical excellence, and leadership development. The abundant literature and research on the importance of mentoring should encourage all members of the profession to establish mentor relationships and mentor programs at each stage of their careers. Each professional nurse has the obligation and privilege to participate in the mentor connection.

REFERENCES

Alleman, E. (1987). *Alleman mentoring scales questionnaire, Form A.* (Available from Leadership Development Consultants, Inc., Mentor, OH.)

Alvarez, A., & Abriam-Yago, K. (1993). Mentoring undergraduate ethnic-minority students: A strategy for retention. *Journal of Nursing Education, 32*(5), 230–232.

American Nurses Association. (1980). *Directory of nurses with doctoral degrees.* Kansas City, MO: Author.

Andersen, S. L. (1989). The nurse advocate project: A strategy to retain new graduates. *Journal of Nursing Administration, 19*(12), 22–26.

Astin, A. W. (1990). Educational assessment and educational equity. *American Journal of Education, 98,* 458–478

Atkins, S., & Williams, A. (1995). Registered nurses' experiences of mentoring undergraduate nursing students. *Journal of Advanced Nursing, 21,* 1006–1015.

Atwood, A. H. (1979). The mentor in clinical practice. *Nursing Outlook, 27,* 714–717.

Baldwin, D., & Wold, J. (1993). Students from disadvantaged backgrounds: Satisfaction with a mentor-protégé relationship. *Journal of Nursing Education, 32*(5), 225–226.

Bandura, A. (1977). *Social learning theory.* Englewood Cliffs, NJ: Prentice Hall.

Bellinger, S. R., & McCloskey, J. C. (1992). Are preceptors for orientation of new nurses effective? *Journal of Professional Nursing, 8*(6), 321–327.

Booth, R. Z. (1992). *The dean's role in organizational assessment and development.* Washington, DC: American Association of Colleges of Nursing.

Butler, M. J. (1989). Mentoring and scholarly productivity in nursing faculty (Doctoral dissertation, West Virginia University, 1989). *Dissertation Abstracts International, 51,* 691A.

Butts, B. J., & Witmer, D. M. (1992). New graduates: What does my manager expect? *Nursing Management, 23*(8), 46–48.

Cahill, M. G., & Kelly, J. J. (1989). A mentor program for nursing majors. *Journal of Nursing Education, 28*(1), 40–44.

Carey, S. J., & Campbell, S. T. (1994). Preceptor, mentor, and sponsor roles: Creative strategies for nurse retention. *Journal of Nursing Administration, 24*(12), 39–48.

Collins, E., & Scott, P. (1978). Everyone who makes it has a mentor. *Harvard Business Review, 56*(4), 89–101.

Creamer, E. G. (1996). The scholarly productivity of women academics. *Initiatives, 57*(4), 1–9.

Daly, A. M., & Jones, T. (1988). An independent study in conjunction with a sophomore nursing course. *Journal of Nursing Education, 27*(5), 231–232.

Davidhizar, R. E. (1988). Mentoring in doctoral education. *Journal of Advanced Nursing, 13,* 775–781.

Dufault, M.A. (1990). Personal and work-milieu resources as variables associated with role mastery in the novice nurse. *The Journal of Continuing Education in Nursing, 21*(2), 73–78.

Erikson, E. (1963). *Childhood and society* (3rd ed.). New York: Norton.

Erikson, E. (1968). *Identity: Youth and crisis.* New York: Norton.

Fagan, M. M., & Fagan, P. D. (1983). Mentoring among nurses. *Nursing & Health Care, 4,* 77–82.

Fields, W. (1991). Mentoring in nursing: A historical approach. *Nursing Outlook, 39,* 257–261.

Flanagan, J. C. (1954). The critical incident technique. *Psychological Bulletin, 51,* 327–359.

Gaspar, T. (1990). Job satisfaction of chairpersons of nursing departments in academe. (Doctoral dissertation, University of Utah, 1990). *Dissertation Abstracts International, 51,* 1192B.

Gilbert, L. A. (1985). Dimensions of same gender student faculty role model relationship. *Sex Roles, 12,* 111–123.

Gjertsen, M. L. (1992). *The relationship between mentorship and leadership effectiveness among a group of graduate nursing students.* Unpublished master's thesis, Sacred Heart University, Fairfield, CT.

Guilbert, E. K. (1979). Health care work powerlessness scale (revised). In *Instruments for measuring nursing practice and other health care variables* (pp. 37-40). Washington, DC: U.S. Department of Health, Education and Welfare, Public Health Service.

Hanson, C. M., & Hilde, E. (1989). Faculty mentorship: Support for nurse practitioner students and staff within the rural community health setting. *Journal of Community Health Nursing, 6*(2), 73–81.

Hayes, E. (1994). Helping preceptors mentor the next generation of nurse practitioners. *Nurse Practitioner, 19*(6), 62–66.

Heinrich, K. T., & Scherr, M. W. (1994). Peer mentoring for reflective teaching: A model for nurses who teach. *Nurse Educator, 19*(4), 36–41.

Herrick, H. S. (1974). *Relationship of organizational structure to teacher motivation in multi-unit and non-unit elementary schools.* Unpublished doctoral dissertation, University of Wisconsin, Madison.

Huang, C. A., & Lynch, J. (1995). *Mentoring: The Tao of giving and receiving wisdom.* New York: HarperSanFrancisco.

Johnson, B. M. (1979). Faculty satisfaction instrument. In M. Word & M. Felter (Eds.), *Instrument for use in nursing education research* (pp. 161–167). Boulder, CO: Western Interstate Commission for Higher Education.

Johnsrud, L. K. (1991). Mentoring between academic women: The capacity for interdependence. *Initiatives, 54*(2), 7–17.

Jowers, L. T., & Herr, K. (1990). A review of literature on mentor-protégé relationships. In G. M. Clayton & P. A. Baj (Eds.), *Review of research in nursing education* (Vol. 3, 49–77). New York: National League for Nursing.

Kavoosi, M. C. (1992). *Faculty mentoring and administrative support in schools of nursing.* Unpublished doctoral dissertation, Univeristy of Pittsburgh, Pittsburgh.

Kavoosi, M. C., Elman, N. S., & Mauch, J. E. (1995). Faculty mentoring and administrative support in schools of nursing. *Journal of Nursing Education, 34*(9), 419–426.

Laird, N. C. (1992). Professional development perceptions of nurses attending the American Association of Colleges of Nursing (AACN) first executive development series (Doctoral dissertation, George Mason University, 1992). *Dissertation Abstracts International, 53,* 770B.

Lamborn, M. L. (1991). Motivation and job satisfaction of deans of schools of nursing. *Journal of Professional Nursing, 7*(1), 33–40.

Larson, O. M. (1994). Career aspirations to higher leadership positions of nurse faculty middle managers. *Journal of Professional Nursing, 10*(3), 147–153.

Larson, E., Hill, M., & Haller, K. (1993). Clinical application of undergraduate research skills. *Nurse Educator, 18*(6), 31–34.

Levinson, D. (1996). *The season's of a woman's life.* New York: Knopf.

Levinson, D., Darrow, C., Klein, E., Levinson, M., & McKee, B. (1979). *The seasons of a man's life.* New York: Ballantine.

Linc, L. G., & Campbell, J. M. (1995). Role models for research. *Advanced Practice Nurse, 2*(2), 19–21, 24.

Martin, M. L., Tolleson, J., Lakey, K. I., & Moeller, E. (1995). VALOR students: A creative type of preceptorship. *Federal Practitioner, 12*(4), 47–50.

May, K. M., Meleis, A. I., & Winstead-Fry, P. (1982). Mentorship for scholarliness: Opportunities and dilemmas. *Nursing Outlook, 30*(1), 22–28.

Megel, M. E. (1985). New faculty in nursing: Socialization and the role of mentor. *Journal of Nursing Education, 24*(7), 303–306.

Megel, M. E., Langston, N. F., & Creswell, J. W. (1988). Scholarly productivity: A survey of nursing faculty researchers. *Journal of Professional Nursing, 4*(1), 45–54.

Meleis, A. I. (1992). On the way to scholarship: From master's to doctorate. *Journal of Professional Nursing, 8*(6), 328–334.

Meleis, A. I., Hall, J. M., & Stevens, P. E. (1994). Scholarly caring in doctoral nursing education: Promoting diversity and collaborative mentorship. *Image: Journal of Nursing Scholarship, 26*(3), 177–180.

McCloskey, J. C. (1974). Influence of rewards and incentives on staff nurse turnover rate. *Nursing Research, 23*, 239–247.

Miles, M. B., & Huberman, A. M. (1984). *Qualitative data analysis.* Beverly Hills, CA: Sage.

Miller, J. O., & Carey, S. J. (1993). Work role inventory: A guide to job satisfaction. *Nursing Management, 24*(1), 54–62.

National Student Nurses Association. (1996). In support of the promotion, awareness, and development of mentorship programs. *Proceedings from NSNA Annual Convention—New Orleans, LA.* New York: Author.

Nayak, S. (1991). Strategies to support the new nurse in practice. *Journal of Nursing Staff Development, 7*(3), 64–66.

Olson, R. K., & Connelly, L. M. (1995). Mentoring through predoctoral fellowships to enhance research productivity. *Journal of Professional Nursing, 11*(5), 270–275.

Olson, R. K., & Vance, C. V. (1993). *Mentorship in nursing: A collection of research abstracts with selected bibliographies—1977–1992.* Houston: University of Texas Printing Services.

Pappas, A. B. (1988). Professional role conflict and related coping strategies of baccalaureate nursing faculty: A phenomenological study (Doctoral dissertation, Texas Women's University, 1988). *Dissertation Abstracts International, 49,* 4234B.

Pierce, C. A. (1983). *Mentoring, gender and attainment: The professional development of academic psychologist.* Unpublished doctoral dissertation, The University of Texas at Austin.

Powell, S. R. (1990). Mentors in nursing in the university setting (Doctoral dissertation, University of Iowa, 1990). *Dissertation Abstracts International, 51,* 5810B.

Princeton, J. C., & Gaspar, T. M. (1991). First-line administrators in academe: How are they prepared, what do they do, and will they stay in their jobs? *Journal of Professional Nursing, 7*(2), 79–87.

Ramsey, D. E., Thompson, J. C., & Brathwaite, H. (1994). Mentoring: A professional commitment. *Journal of the National Black Nurses Association, 7*(1), 68–76.

Rawl, S. M. (1989). Nursing education administrators: Level of career development and mentoring (Doctoral dissertation, University of Illinois, Chicago, 1989). *Dissertation Abstracts International, 50,* 1857B.

Rawl, S. M., & Peterson, L. M. (1992). Nursing education administrators: Level of career development and mentoring. *Journal of Professional Nursing, 8*(3), 161–169.

Redmond, G. M. (1991). Life and career pathways of deans in nursing programs. *Journal of Professional Nursing, 7*(4), 228–238.

Roche, G. (1979). Much ado about mentors. *Harvard Business Review, 57*(1), 14–16, 20, 24, 26–28.

Rollin, M. J. (1991). The prevalence and characteristics of mentors, protégés, and mentor–protégé relationships among nurse educators (Master's thesis, Duquesne University, 1991). *Master's Abstracts International, 30,* 715.

Schorr, T. M., & Zimmerman, A. (1988). *Making choices taking chances: Nurse leaders tell their stories.* St. Louis: Mosby.

Schwerian, P. (1978). Evaluating the performance of nurses: A multidimensional approach. *Nursing Research, 27,* 347–351.

Schwerin, J., Gaster, K., Krolikowski, J., & Sherman-Justice, D. (1994). Staff nurse leadership and professional growth in the mentor role. *Journal of Nursing Staff Development, 10*(3), 139–144.

Short, J. D. (1997a). Profile of administrators of schools of nursing: Part I Resources for goal achievement. *Journal of Professional Nursing, 13*(1), 7–12.

Short, J. D. (1997b). Profile of administrators of schools of nursing: Part II Mentoring relationships and influence activities. *Journal of Professional Nursing, 13*(1), 13–18.

Smith, P. C., Kendall, L. M., & Hulin, C. L. (1969). *The measurement of satisfaction in work and retirement.* Chicago: Rand McNally.

Spengler, C. D. (1982). Mentor–protégé relationships: A study of career development among female nurse doctorates (Doctoral dissertation, University of Missouri, Columbia, 1982). *Dissertation Abstracts International, 44,* 2113B.

Stogdill, R. M. (1963). *Manual for the leader behavior description questionnaire—Form xii: An experimental revision.* Columbus: Ohio State University.

Taylor, L. J. (1992). A survey of mentor relationships in academe. *Journal of Professional Nursing, 8*(1), 48–55.

Turton, S., & Herriot, S. (1989). Mentoring psychiatric student nurses. *Nursing Times, 85*(36), 70–71.

Valverde, L. A. (1980). Development of ethnic researchers and the education of white researchers. *Educational Researcher, 9*(9), 16–20.

Vance, C. (1977). A group profile of contemporary influentials in American nursing (Doctoral dissertation, Teachers College, Columbia University, 1977). *Dissertation Abstracts International, 38,* 4734B.

Vance, C. N., & Olson, R. K. (1991). Mentorship in nursing. In J. J. Fitzpatrick, R. L. Taunton, & A. K. Jacox (Eds.), *Annual review of nursing research* (Vol. 9, p. 175–200). New York: Springer.

Vance, C. N., & Olson, R. K. (1998). *The mentor connection in nursing.* New York: Springer.

Waters, C. M. (1996). Professional development in nursing research—A culturally diverse postdoctoral experience. *Image: Journal of Nursing Scholarship, 28*(1), 47–50.

Watson, P. G. (1990). Faculty research skills development. *Journal of Allied Health, 19*(1), 25–37.

Wocial, L. D. (1995). The role of mentors in promoting integrity and preventing scientific misconduct in nursing research. *Journal of Professional Nursing, 11*(5), 276–280.

Yoder, L. H. (1990). Mentoring: A concept analysis. *Nursing Administration Quarterly, 15*(1), 9–19.

Zimmerman, L., & Yeaworth, R. (1986). Factors influencing career success in nursing. *Research in Nursing & Health, 9,* 179–185.

Chapter 3

Teaching Psychomotor Nursing Skills in Simulated Learning Labs: A Critical Review of the Literature

DONNA JO MIRACLE, RN, C, MSN

INTRODUCTION

Methods of simulated design have become the standard by which psychomotor nursing skills are taught to nursing students and novice clinicians; however, these strategies continue to be implemented without a theoretical or empirical basis for decisions regarding learning methods. If research is to guide practice, teaching methods must be based on research findings. The purpose of this chapter is to summarize research findings on educational strategies and innovations for teaching psychomotor nursing skills to nursing students. Past and current strategies in teaching psychomotor skills are reviewed.

Historically, psychomotor skills were taught during on-the-job training in the clinical setting. The movement of nursing education from apprenticeship to colleges and universities changed the setting for teaching psychomotor skills. Simulated design became the method for teaching psychomotor skills, with various teaching strategies incorporating multimedia (audiocassette, videotape, interactive video, and computer-assisted instruction), demonstration/return demonstration, learning modules, faculty-assisted versus self-instruction, and mental imagery. The demand on time resources along with patients' perceptions of the importance of psychomotor skills has raised awareness among nurse educators regarding methods for teaching these skills. Changes in health care delivery have increased the time that nurse clinicians spend performing psychomotor skills. This has come about with little mentoring for the development of these skills. Patients have reported that the efficiency as well as proficiency with which the practitioner performs technical skills can be anxiety producing or reducing (Bjork, 1995).

Teaching psychomotor skills is central to many curricular issues in nursing education. The changing health care environment limits opportunities to practice psychomotor skills with faculty supervision. Shortened hospital stays, high patient acuity, and a shift to home care present new challenges for teaching psychomotor skills to the beginning nursing student.

Richardson (1969) described psychomotor skills as manipulative skills that require the learner to perceive and coordinate sensory stimuli to complete purposeful movements. There are three types of psychomotor skills—fine, manual, and gross—all of which are important in designing and implementing optimum learning situations. The development of psychomotor skills is a complex process, and individual differences are important considerations in the learning of these skills. These differences include manual dexterity, attitude, motivation, confidence, kinesthetic awareness, intelligence, and/or age of the learners (de Tornyay & Thompson, 1987).

Methods

Automated and manual bibliographic searches were conducted to identify research studies for analysis using the keywords *psychomotor, psychomotor performance, motor skills, psychomotor skills, technologies, teaching skills, nursing skills, and learning resource laboratory.* Databases from 1982 to 1998 were searched for articles regarding psychomotor skills in nursing education. The sources searched included the Cumulative Index to Nursing and Allied Health Literature (CINAHL), Medline, textbooks, and abstracts from recent conferences. The Educational Resources Information Center (ERIC) database was searched; however, no research on nursing skills development was identified. To be included in this review, the research needed to focus on psychomotor skills and represent empirical studies within a nursing simulated laboratory or clinical setting.

Twenty-five articles met these criteria and provided information used to evaluate the published literature and to identify gaps in the research. The articles were analyzed for key themes and categorized using content analysis procedures. This technique provided a systematic means to identify the themes and place the articles into categories. To perform the content analysis, each title was reviewed for individual words or word combinations. In some cases, more than one theme was identified from a single article. In addition, the themes were verified through consultation with two nurse educators with expertise in instructional materials in the nursing laboratory. The themes that emerged with greatest frequency were used as key themes for categorization. The resulting categories were mutually exclusive. In addition to these research reports, a number of anecdotal and theoretical articles were used to provide definitions and background on the topic.

Themes

The resulting themes were essential skills and competency, teaching strategies (performance checklists, mental imagery, simulation, multimedia), educational setting, and learner variables. Table 3–1 presents the frequency of each theme found in the 25 studies. Less frequent topics included the changing health care environment, role of the faculty, student outcome/satisfaction, and future changes and challenges in nursing education. The key themes are used as organizers in this review with the importance for nursing education discussed with each topic (see Table 3–2).

TABLE 3–1.
Content Analysis of 25 Research Reports

Themes	Frequency of Theme
Essential skills	4
Competency level	2
Teaching strategies	13
Educational setting	5
Learner variables	1

Note. Some reports contained more than one theme.

TABLE 3–2.

Summary of Literature on Teaching Psychomotor Nursing Skills in the Learning Laboratory and Clinical Setting

Study/Anecdotal Report	Purpose/Design	Major Results
Essential Skills		
	Skills and Competency	
Sweeney et al. (1982)	Investigate the priority that baccalaureate nursing faculty placed on teaching psychomotor skills in an undergraduate program. Quasi-experimental design. Sample: 15 baccalaureate program faculty.	The study found that essential skills were not clearly defined. Faculty did not see some of the more commonly expected skills as essential. Limitations: small sample size.
Sweeney and Regan (1982)	Document responses of baccalaureate graduates in rating the relative importance of a number of psychomotor skills. This expanded a previous study that compared nursing administrators and nurse educators in determining essential skills for nursing students. Comparative experimental design. Sample: 15 baccalaureate program faculty.	The study found discrepancies among the expectations of faculty, nursing service personnel, and recent baccalaureate graduates with regard to essential skills. Limitations: small sample size.
Kieffer (1984)	Describe a method using data from the clinical setting to assist nurse educators in selecting technical nursing skills to teach for competency within the basic nursing program. Pilot project. Sample: 54 staff nurses.	The project helped faculty examine skills placement. This was helpful in deciding which skills to select and which to eliminate from the program. Limitations: small sample size.
Anderson et al. (1985)	Develop a framework to implement psychomotor component in a nursing curriculum. Description of psychomotor skills in a nursing curriculum.	The authors formulated a list of psychomotor skills and leveled these skills with the appropriate nursing theory and practicum courses. Limitations: study design, anecdotal report.

TABLE 3–2.
*Summary of Literature on Teaching Psychomotor Nursing Skills
in the Learning Laboratory and Clinical Setting (Continued)*

Study/Anecdotal Report	Purpose/Design	Major Results
Alavi et al. (1991)	Describe a process of determining the psychomotor skills to be taught in an undergraduate nursing program. Data collection/frequency tabulation. Sample: 59 clinical agencies.	A psychomotor skills grid was developed to be used with teaching technological skills as well as the designated level of competency. Limitations: Small sample size, study design.
Studdy et al. (1984)	Describe the development of a multidisciplinary skills center. Description of a model for teaching clinical skills.	A two-part report identified necessary skills to be acquired in a multidisciplinary skills laboratory and the level of performance at various stages. Limitations: study design, anecdotal report.
Competency Level		
Hallal & Welsh (1984)	Describe the implementation of a learning laboratory in a baccalaureate nursing program and evaluate the effectiveness. Comparative study. Sample: 36 nursing students.	The two most critical factors for success in the competency laboratory were student accountability and efficient time scheduling. Limitations: small sample size.
del Bueno et al. (1987)	Describe the development of a competency-based assessment center. Descriptive study. Sample: 21 Intensive care nurses.	The center provided a cost-effective alternative to the traditional way in which decisions were made about what individuals need to become competent performers. There was a 20–35% reduction in nonproductivity costs of competency development reported. Limitations: small sample size, study design.
Garcia (1988)	Compare the expectations of head nurses and nursing instructors on psychomotor skill competencies of entry-level professional nurses. Sample: unknown	Expectations for psychomotor skill competencies of entry-level professional nurses were significantly different between head nurses and nursing instructors. Limitations: unpublished manuscript.

TABLE 3-2.
Summary of Literature on Teaching Psychomotor Nursing Skills in the Learning Laboratory and Clinical Setting (Continued)

Study/Anecdotal Report	Purpose/Design	Major Results
Hodson et al. (1988)	Report on the development and implementation of a multimedia module to guide the nursing student through a clinical day simulation. Descriptive study. Sample: 80 sophomore baccaulareate nursing students.	Successful implementation of the module was reported. The students had a well-defined self-instructional procedure for the simulation practice and evaluation experience. Limitations: Small sample size, study design.
Miller (1989)	Survey comparing the perceptions of nursing faculty and nursing service personnel on psychomotor competencies for graduate baccalaureate nurses. Sample: unknown.	Nursing faculty rated student performance of psychomotor skills at a higher level of competence than nursing service personnel. Limitations: Unpublished manuscript.
	Teaching Strategies	
Performance Checklist		
McCaffrey (1978)	Describe the development of a performance checklist for evaluation of psychomotor skills. Anecdotal report.	A performance checklist was developed for neurological examination. The authors described the tool as "effective and efficient for teaching and evaluating." Limitations: no study design.
Mooney (1993)	Develop a performance checklist that would demonstrate how complicated such a tool can be for a student. Anecdotal report.	Findings suggested that the skilled nurse knows how to perform tasks presented on a checklist, but learners find the checklist itself to be a source of anxiety. Limitations: no study design.

TABLE 3–2.
Summary of Literature on Teaching Psychomotor Nursing Skills in the Learning Laboratory and Clinical Setting (Continued)

Study/Anecdotal Report	Purpose/Design	Major Results
Mental Imagery		
Eaton & Evans (1986)	Examine imagery ability in improving methods of teaching psychomotor nursing skills. Experimental design. Sample: 80 nursing students.	The imaging ability of low imagers was enhanced after two brief practice sessions. Limitations: Small sample size.
Bachman (1990)	Explore the usefulness of mental imagery as a technique for practicing psychomotor nursing skills. Experimental design. Sample: 22 registered nurses.	Subjects were able to clearly perceive a specific psychomotor skill using mental imagery. No significant differences were noted in the performance of the study and control groups. Limitations: small sample size.
Smith (1992)	Compare two cognitive strategies (Vee heuristics and concept maps) that identify connections between scientific theory and practice. Quasi-experimental design. Sample: 42 junior-level nursing students.	Students using Vee heuristics and concept maps, rather than traditional modes, were significantly better able to identify scientific principles to justify specific steps of a nursing skill. Limitations: small sample size.
Bucher (1993)	Explore the interactive effects of imagery skills and various combinations of physical and mental practice on learning a skill. Experimental design. Sample: 60 nursing students.	A significant main effect was obtained for practice condition. It was suggested that this study be replicated with larger samples of male students, students from different types of nursing programs, and nontraditional students. Limitations: Instrumentation issues, small number of subjects in each treatment cell.
Doheney (1993)	Determine whether mental imaging practice for nursing students affected learning and performance of an intramuscular injection. Experimental design. Sample: 95 sophomore baccalaureate nursing students.	Findings suggested that the use of mental practice does affect learning and performance of motor skills. Limitations: small sample size.

TABLE 3–2.
Summary of Literature on Teaching Psychomotor Nursing Skills in the Learning Laboratory and Clinical Setting (Continued)

Study/Anecdotal Report	Purpose/Design	Major Results
Simulation		
Cowan & Wiens (1986)	Develop a mock hospital for a preclinical laboratory experience. This was designed to decrease anxiety and increase student competence in communication and psychomotor skills. Descriptive study. Sample: nursing students.	Evaluation forms were completed by both students and volunteers assisting with the simulation. Both groups rated this experience as important for the practice of skills in a supervised situation. Limitations: sample size not reported, study design.
McDonald (1987)	Describe teaching methods used in a senior clinical course simulation exercise. Anecdotal report.	Described a teaching method for nursing interventions in client situations that encompassed multiple problems. Limitations: No study design.
Lowdermilk and Fishel (1991)	Study the use of computer simulations as a strategy to evaluate clinical decision-making skills of baccalaureate nursing students. Quasi-experimental design. Sample: 64 senior baccalaureate nursing students.	No difference was found between students who completed the full computer-assisted instruction series and those who did not. Limitations: small sample size, study design.
Erler & Rudman (1993)	Determine the effect of a campus critical care simulation on anxiety of nursing students in the clinical intensive care unit. Quasi-experimental, pretest-posttest design. Sample: 50 junior-level baccalaureate nursing students.	Findings indicated that familiarity with psychomotor skills is not sufficient to decrease anxiety in the critical care clinical setting. Limitations: small sample size, convenience sample, lack of control over personal variables that contribute to anxiety.
Bradbury-Golas & Carson (1994)	Describe the development and implementation of a successful nursing skills fair. Descriptive study. Sample: 150 staff nurses.	A nursing skills fair was conducted and reported as successful in offering an approach for learner independence. The fair was especially important given the differing levels of knowledge, development, and skill throughout an institution. Limitations: study design.

TABLE 3-2.
Summary of Literature on Teaching Psychomotor Nursing Skills in the Learning Laboratory and Clinical Setting (Continued)

Study/Anecdotal Report	Purpose/Design	Major Results
White (1995)	Compare the use of the problem-solving process with computer simulations and actual patients. Quasi-experimental design. Sample: 16 nursing students.	Criterion validity of the simulations was established. Limitations: small sample size.
Multimedia		
Love et al. (1989)	Compare the effectiveness of teaching psychomotor skills in a structured laboratory setting with self-taught modules. Randomized control trial. Sample: 77 sophomore baccalaureate nursing students.	Findings substantiated the hypothesis of no difference between psychomotor skill performance of students who learn in a self-directed manner and those taught in a structured clinical laboratory. Limitations: small sample size.
Brigham et al. (1991)	Report on the development, implementation, and evaluation of a multimedia asepsis module incorporating universal precautions. Descriptive study. Sample: 191 nursing students.	Faculty supervised 4-station participatory learning modules. Student evaluations were positive. Limitations: study design.
Urick & Bond (1994)	Report on the conversion of an outdated media center into a computer laboratory. Anecdotal report.	The conversion was successful. All basic skills are now taught by self-instructional methodology using multimedia as a result of this teaching design. Limitations: no study design.
Educational Setting		
Kolb and Shugart (1984)	Examine the advantages and disadvantages of utilizing simulation for evaluation. Descriptive study. Sample: none.	A planning guide was developed to be used with simulation in the evaluation process. Criteria for evaluation were established. Limitations: no study design.

TABLE 3–2.
Summary of Literature on Teaching Psychomotor Nursing Skills in the Learning Laboratory and Clinical Setting (Continued)

Study/Anecdotal Report	Purpose/Design	Major Results
Gomez & Gomez (1987)	Investigate practice conditions when learning a psychomotor skill in a baccalaureate program in nursing. Quasi-experimental design. Sample: 63 baccalaureate nursing students.	Practice of an open psychomotor skill was more effective and more meaningful in the patient care setting than the school laboratory. Limitations: small sample size.
Elliott et al. (1982)	Discover the emphasis that psychomotor skill learning receives in undergraduate nursing programs and determine the extent to which nursing curricula reflect current research and knowledge in this area. Descriptive study. Sample: 38 schools of nursing in the United States and Canada.	Three trends were identified: 1. Trend toward decreasing availability of adequate clinical facilities for students to practice skill learning. 2. Increasing awareness of human rights issues on the part of both consumer and health care professional. 3. Expanding availability of educational hardware and software as well as increased use of audiovisual materials, learning packages, computer-assisted instruction, and closed-circuit TV. Limitations: small sample size, study design.
Pelletier (1995)	Study how diploma-prepared registered nurses from tertiary institutions perceived their ability to handle technical equipment in the workplace. Correlational design. Sample: 245 diploma-registered nurses.	No significant relationship was found between the frequency of use of specific items of clinical equipment and whether those items caused the nurse concern in practice. No significant relationship was found between the frequency of use of an item and whether participants believed that competence in relation to that item should be acquired in relation to that item prior to graduation. Limitations: further testing needed on questionnaire and replication of study.

TABLE 3-2.
Summary of Literature on Teaching Psychomotor Nursing Skills in the Learning Laboratory and Clinical Setting (Continued)

Study/Anecdotal Report	Purpose/Design	Major Results
Learner Variables		
Goldsmith (1984)	Investigate the interactions between three learner variables associated with learning a psychomotor nursing task. Quasi-experimental design. Sample: 55 female baccalaureate nursing students.	The authors suggested that the effect of these variables on learning be studied over a longer period of time. Limitations: small sample size, study design.
Review of Literature		
Thompson & Crutchlow (1993)	Critical review of the literature to research learning styles published in education and nursing literature.	Concept was extensively researched in general education; however, limited research was found in nursing literature.
Oermann (1990)	Explore the process of psychomotor skill development.	Psychomotor skills were defined and guidelines addressed for beginning skill development. Theoretical concepts were gathered.

SKILLS AND COMPETENCY

Nature of Psychomotor Skills

When psychomotor skills are taught the movement dimension is emphasized, but in practice performance, cognitive/affective dimensions must be integrated with the motor dimension. Oermann (1990) explored the process of psychomotor skill development and developed guidelines for teaching motor skills. Psychomotor skills were classified into three categories: gross motor skills (tasks involving large muscles and movement), manual skills (manipulative, repetitive tasks), and fine motor skills (precision-oriented tasks). The author suggested that the nurse develops skill in performance through practice. Practice provides the means through which smooth, coordinated movement can be developed. Oermann (1990) emphasized the importance of separating the cognitive and affective dimensions of the skill from the motor dimension during the teaching process. One guideline that Oermann set forth was that discussion of principles underlying the skill, the rationale for its use, and other theoretical aspects should be separated from skill instruction to allow the nurse to focus on the movements themselves. Another guideline addressed beginning skill learning. Oermann reported that demonstration of the procedure is important, for at this point learners observe the skill, develop a mental image of the performance, and subsequently practice it until their own performances are congruent with the mental image. Furthermore, feedback from the teacher is important to skill development so the learner can adjust his or her performance to refine movements, correct errors, and improve accuracy and speed (Oermann, 1990).

Essential Skills

What essential skills should be included in a curriculum designed for the beginning student in the laboratory setting? Sweeney, Hedstrom, and O'Malley (1982) investigated the priority that baccalaureate nursing faculty placed on teaching psychomotor skills in an undergraduate program. Subjects included 15 randomly selected faculty, who rated 291 psychomotor skills as essential (every student needs to perform this procedure safely prior to graduation), bonus (it would be nice if every student had the opportunity to perform this procedure, but not essential), graduate (complex procedure that needs greater understanding, guidance, and practice than can be provided in an undergraduate nursing program), and nonnursing (should be performed by personnel other than nurses). The authors found that 121 skills were rated essential by 90% of faculty. No skills reached 90% agreement in the graduate or nonnursing categories, while four skills were classified as bonus by the entire group. The authors noted lack of faculty agreement regarding the importance of teaching over half of the skills. The study found that essential skills were not clearly defined (especially in the more technically complex areas of nursing skills) and faculty did not deem some of the more commonly expected skills as essential.

Further study was conducted by Sweeney and Regan (1982) to identify the importance placed on teaching specific psychomotor skills in a baccalaureate program by three contrasting groups of nurses: nurse educators, nursing service personnel, and new baccalaureate graduates. Samples of 15 subjects were obtained for each of the three categories. A list of 291 psychomotor skills (suggested in the literature for inclusion in a baccalaureate curriculum) were compiled, and subjects were asked to sort these skills into four categories. The four categories developed and defined by Sweeney et al. (1982) (essential, bonus, graduate, and nonnursing) were used. The authors found that all three groups basically agreed on slightly more than half of the skills. Essential skills totaled 131, and bonus skills 17; one skill was listed as nonnursing and two skills were split evenly between the essential and bonus categories. Complete agreement was obtained on only 10% of the entire list. The authors found no agreement on the graduate-level skills. A review of the findings from each group demonstrated that nursing service personnel hold the most diverse opinions concerning the importance of psychomotor skills. A larger number of skills, particularly those of a technically complex nature, were designated essential by that group. The authors suggested that the findings indicated nursing service personnel expect new graduates to enter the hospital setting with a wider repertoire of skills than do faculty or new graduates.

The studies by Sweeney et al. (1982) and Sweeney and Regan (1982) indicate a need to identify specific psychomotor skills that are important and essential for baccalaureate students to perform before graduation. Lack of consensus within a program may lead to confusion about the expected skill performance, which is amplified later when the graduate encounters employer and patient expectations. The authors suggested further investigation to determine the most efficient manner in which these skills can be taught and in what type of setting (laboratory, clinical, or both).

Kieffer (1984) conducted a pilot project using data from clinical settings to assist nurse educators in selecting technical nursing skills to teach for competency within the basic nursing program. The project was based on the assumptions that frequency and importance of technical skills vary depending upon the setting and client population; new graduates should be competent to perform those technical skills identified as most frequent as well as most important in client care; and essential skills can be determined by polling nurses practicing in clinical areas where new graduates are most often employed. The authors developed a questionnaire that was administered to nurses from 16 hospitals with a sample of 54 obtained. Skills ranking in the top 25% included (a) assessment of vital signs; (b) assisting with elimination, hygiene, and asepsis; (c) medication administration; and (d) use of sterile technique. Keifter reported that skills ranked in the upper half of the midrange were consistent with skills commonly taught. Results of the study were used by the associate degree faculty to examine skills taught in the program. The rankings reinforced the continued teaching of skills currently included and gave direction for adding or deleting other specific skills. Faculty decided that skills identified in the top 25% frequency or importance for all clinical groups combined would be taught for competency. Keiffer (1984) recommended further refinement of the research instrument and data collection process. A larger sample would increase generalizability, and replication should address reliability and internal consistency of the findings.

From a different perspective, Anderson, Conklin, Watson, Hirst, and Hoffman (1985) developed a framework for implementating the psychomotor component in a nursing curriculum. Once the framework for the psychomotor domain was developed, essential nursing skills were identified. The authors defined essential nursing skills as those nursing activities deemed necessary to carry out the nursing process. A list of essential psychomotor skills was formulated using a review of current literature and a survey from nursing school faculty. The selected psychomotor skills were then leveled with the appropriate nursing theory and practicum courses throughout the nursing program. Leveling provided for minimum acceptable achievement based on Dave's (Dave, 1970) taxonomy (organization of behaviors that require neuromuscular coordination). The organization of behaviors are categorized through five processes: imitation, manipulation, precision, articulation, and naturalization. In conjunction with this work, testing was designed to assess acquisition of essential psychomotor skills at either the level of precision or the level of articulation in the simulated laboratory setting. Thus, the student would perform at the designated achievement level prior to performing a psychomotor skill involving an actual client. The authors reported five benefits to the development of the psychomotor domain: (a) helping learners develop and refine psychomotor skills within a supervised environment, (b) provision of a safe and practical experience for students in a controlled learning environment where experiences can be organized and predictable, (c) availability of faculty members with clearly defined guidelines on how to teach students psychomotor skills, (d) graduation of competent nurses with skills fundamental to the practice of nursing, and (e) a strengthened curriculum because of a more fully developed psychomotor domain to meet students' learning needs (Anderson, Conklin, Watson, Hirst, & Hoffman, 1985).

In comparison, Alavi, Loh, and Reilly (1991) studied the psychomotor skills that should be incorporated into the nursing curriculum and to what degree of competency each skill should be achieved. The study included 59 faculty members. A psychomotor skills grid served as a guide for teaching the psychomotor domain of this undergraduate nursing curriculum. Decisions about the psychomotor skills to be included in this psychomotor grid and the level of competency that students should be expected to reach during their educational program were selected (by the faculty) from those that were considered integral to comprehensive nursing practice. The selection process by faculty involved two criteria: frequency of use within nursing practice, and the opportunity available for practice experience so the desired level of competency could be achieved. The psychomotor skills categories were fundamental skills, general therapeutic and diagnostic skills, and specialized therapeutic and diagnostic skills. Data for each item were placed into categories according to degree of usage. Skills with a total frequency rating of 65% were included in the educational program. The fundamental skills were mobilization of patient, range of motion, body mechanics, lifting, shower-ing, bed-bathing, mouth care, hair care, nail care, positioning, pressure area care, hand washing, bed making, feeding a patient, assisting with bedpan/urinal/commode, and measuring temperature, pulse, respiration, blood pressure, and weight/height. The general therapeutic and diagnostic procedures included inspection, auscultation (bowel sounds, heart sounds, respiratory sounds), palpa-tion, percussion, ear/nose/throat assessment, neurological assessment, inte-grated physical assessment, specimen collection, administration of medications, bandage application, surgical asepsis, wound drainage, removal of sutures/sta-ples, intravenous therapy, isolation techniques, catheterization, urinalysis, cleans-ing enema, suppositories, and hot/cold applications. The special therapeutic and diagnostic measures were oxygen therapy, oropharyngeal suction, tracheostomy suction, stoma therapy, nasogastric tube, eye toilets, eye irrigation, eye drops, nose drops, orthopedic applications, baby bath, assessment of neonate, assess-ment of child's physical development, measurement of central venous pressure, intercostal catheter care, and cardiopulmonary resuscitation. Faculty judgment determined the inclusion of particular skills that did not meet the criteria. Four skills (bed-bathing, axillary temperature measurement, sterile gloving, and wound drainage) were subjected to further discrimination because they had a lower than 65% frequency but had a 70% or higher frequency rating in the clinical setting (Alavi et al., 1991). The levels of seven skills were raised contrary to the criteria of data indications. The faculty decided six of these skills (inspection, aus-cultation of bowel sounds, normal heart sounds, respiratory sounds, palpation, and percussion) were essential because they related to physical assessment. The seventh skill (body mechanics) was deemed by the faculty to be a fundamental skill underlying nursing practice. Intravenous medication had a high frequency total but faculty decided this skill would only be taught in the skills laboratory, because practice experience in the clinical setting was limited. Six skills were elim-inated from the undergraduate teaching program when data indicated they were infrequently used or highly specialized. These skills were inhalation therapy, blad-der washout, peritoneal dialysis, bowel washout, ear drops, and traction. Five levels of competency were identified: imitation, manipulation, precision, articu-lation, and naturalization. Two criteria were used in making a decision about the level to be attained: acceptance of the psychomotor skill within the broad scope of nursing practice, and opportunities available to the student to practice the skill in the clinical setting. Alavi et al., (1991) recommended that levels identified in the grid are minimum levels to be attained by students. The level to be attained for each skill was determined by what all students in the undergraduate program could reasonably achieve. Higher levels of achievement were expected once clin-ical experience was available.

Following the work of Alvai and associates (1991), Studdy, Nicol, and Fox-Hiley (1994) published a two-part report relating to teaching and learning clin-ical skills. Part I described the development of a multidisciplinary skills center, and Part II described the development of a teaching model and schedule of skills. The changing health care environment stimulated medical and nursing staff to explore approaches to teaching and learning psychomotor skills. To meet these changes, a consortium developed a clinical skills learning facility that focused on learning and assessment of clinical and communication skills in a multidisciplinary environment (Studdy et al., 1994). A multidisciplinary environment (nursing students, medical students, and qualified staff from all health care disciplines) was chosen as part of the consortium for a number of reasons. First, the resources required for a skills center are scarce, expensive, and unlikely to be found in one institution. Second and equally important was the belief that health care depends on teamwork and the key to success is mutual respect and understanding among team members. Finally, multidisciplinary collaboration provides the opportunity for further developments as well as the possibility of joint research. Studdy et al. (1994) identified skills to be acquired and the level of performance at specific stages throughout the project.

Nurse educators continue to debate the essential skills to be included in the educational curriculum. The rapidly changing health care environment, along with technological advances, places increasing demands on nursing education to provide a graduate who is a skilled practitioner as well as cognitively prepared. Including clinical agencies in the data collection provided graduate nurses with skills conforming to current nursing practice (Alavi et al., 1991). The collaboration of education with clinical facilities is an essential ingredient in preparing graduates to meet these demands.

Competency Level

Nursing students must perform psychomotor skills at a minimal competency level to ensure safety to clients. Within this context, Corcoran (1977) looked at the ethical questions involved in using a service setting as a learning laboratory. Questions were raised regarding methodologies for developing and integrating intellectual abilities, attitudes, values, and technical skills necessary for professional practice. Throughout the nursing literature there is discussion regarding the role of faculty in teaching skills and the outcomes of teaching the skills (Corcoran, 1977; Field, Gallman, Nicholson, & Dreher, 1984; Gudmundsen, 1975; Stern, 1988; Woolley, 1977). Woolley (1977) traced skill controversy in nursing education from decades of practice on patients to decades of practice on mannequins. The controversy centered around several questions: Should psychomotor skills be taught and evaluated in the campus laboratory or the clinical setting? Which skills should be taught in the laboratory versus the clinical setting? How are critical decision making and problem solving included with psychomotor skill teaching and evaluation? How can a conceptual framework link knowledge of clinical skills with skill performance? The debate and discussions continued as technology integration and research level advanced in nursing. According to Hodson, Brigham, Hanson, and Armstrong (1988), the psychomotor skill controversy debate has resulted in curricular variations and has stimulated investigation to identify the most appropriate instructional approach for teaching psychomotor skills. Stern (1988) reported that lower priority was being given to the more traditional clinical nursing skills and higher priority given to computer literacy and nursing theory in curricula. Bevis and Clayton (1988) and Bolton (1984) found that nursing programs (especially at the baccalaureate level) emphasized liberal arts and basic science courses with cognitive, communication, research, and psychosocial skills over the teaching of psychomotor skills. The emphasis on these components is intended to produce creativity, critical thinking, and individualized client care.

The Dreyfus model (1980) described the process of skill acquisition as five levels of proficiency: novice, advanced beginner, competent, proficient, and expert. Benner (1984) used the Dreyfus model to describe the process of competency development in nurses. Benner (1984) described novices as persons who have had no experience of the situations in which they are expected to perform. Advanced beginners were described as those who demonstrate marginally acceptable performance and relate with recurring meaningful situational components. Competent students were those who begin to see their action in terms of deliberately planned, long-range goals with clear priorities. The proficient students were described as those who perceive situations as wholes and whose performance was guided by maxims and keen perception. Experts were defined as those who have an enormous background of experience with an intuitive grasp of each situation. Experts were further defined as those who zero in on the problem and are fluid, flexible, and highly proficient. Benner (1984) described nurses who graduate from educational programs on a continuum from advanced beginner to competent performer. According to Benner (1984), the nurse's competence develops as clinical experiences provide opportunity to incorporate knowledge into performance.

A comparative study evaluating the effectiveness of the "competency laboratory" was conducted by Hallal and Welsh (1984). In the laboratory, students could practice and were tested on a core of basic nursing skills, including handwashing, assessing vital signs, bathing, oral hygiene, body mechanics, and bedmaking. The effectiveness of the laboratory was evaluated by comparing the results of a questionnaire administered to students before and after the competency laboratory experience. The study found the two most critical factors for success in the competency laboratory were student accountability and efficient time scheduling. In another study, del Bueno, Weeks, and Brown-Stewart (1987) described the development of a competency-based assessment center. The assessment center was developed to evaluate competent performance and productivity in simulated job situations. The Performance Based Development System (PBDS) Assessment Center focused on clinical assessment. Criteria-based performance standards for a clinical nurse were developed using a construct of three overlapping circles (technical skills, interpersonal relation skills, and critical thinking). Clinical experts developed a set of critical behaviors or criteria for each high-frequency, high-risk procedure. This set of criteria (criterion checklist) was used to evaluate observed performance. Inter-rater reliabilility was established by clinical experts for each criterion checklist, although the checklist was not included in the report. In the first two months of operation, 21 nurses who were hired for or transferred to intensive care units used the assessment center. This group included new graduates, nurses experienced in medical–surgical nursing, and experienced intensive care nurses. Bueno et al. (1987) reported that implementing a clinical assessment center was a valid, reliable method for making objective decisions about nurses' abilities to perform skills. The authors found a cost-effective alternative to the traditional way in which decisions are made about what individuals need to become competent performers. There was a 20%–35% reduction in nonproductivity costs for competency development.

Educators and clinicians may have different expectations of skill competence in new graduates. The minimal research on skill competence, assessments, and expectations indicates disparate opinions between these two groups. A comparison study was conducted by Garcia (1988) of head nurses' and nursing instructors' expectations on psychomotor skill competencies of entry-level professional nurses from associate degree, diploma, and baccalaureate degree nursing programs. Garcia found that head nurses and instructors had significantly different expectations for psychomotor skill competencies of entry-level professional nurses. Data analysis led to a compilation of lists of psychomotor skills for which expectations differed significantly. Garcia (1988) recommended increased articulation between education and service, careful examination of nursing roles, responsibilities, and job descriptions in the acute care setting, and curriculum reform.

Miller (1989) compared the perceptions of nursing faculty and nursing service personnel on psychomotor competencies for graduate baccalaureate nurses. Miller found the two groups did not have the same perceptions of competency or complexity of psychomotor skills. Nursing faculty rated the students' performance of psychomotor skills in the categories of nursing procedures at a higher level of competence than did nursing service personnel (Miller, 1989). The information found in these studies is valuable in providing direction for future research projects. However, the reports by Garcia (1988) and Miller (1989) were unpublished manuscripts and therefore add limited information to the body of nursing knowledge.

The level of competency at which psychomotor nursing skills should be achieved remains in a state of transition. As nursing care continues to shift to the outpatient and home setting, the demand for the graduate to be educated for independent practice is increasing. This shift in setting requires the graduate to perform psychomotor nursing skills without support personnel immediately accessible. The streamlining of psychomotor skills and the limited time frame in which the student can work toward a level of competence in the educational setting may leave gaps in the nursing student's skills. These issues become particularly important when considering the independent setting in which these skills will be practiced and the level of decision making required.

TEACHING STRATEGIES

Educators have used a variety of strategies in teaching psychomotor skills. These include performance checklists, simulation, demonstrations, verbal feedback, self-instruction, faculty-assisted instruction, visual aids, and mental rehearsal. Several studies have examined the use of multimedia in the laboratory. Generally, limited attention has been directed toward teaching strategies within the psychomotor domain.

Performance Checklists

Checklists are frequently used to evaluate psychomotor skills. Each behavior the learner needs to demonstrate for successful performance of a procedure is included in a checklist. Two anecdotal accounts found in the nursing literature describe the development of a performance checklist for evaluation of psychomotor skills. No research reports were found.

A performance checklist for neurological examination was developed by McCaffrey (1978), who concluded that the checklist was an "effective and efficient tool for teaching and evaluating" (p. 13). The evaluation was based on the premise of self-paced learning, immediate feedback, and reinforcement of performance. From a contrary viewpoint, Mooney (1993) developed a humorous checklist to demonstrate the complexity of a performance checklist and the stress it provokes within an individual. By developing of a performance checklist on the act of juggling, the author used humor to demonstrate how "absurd, complicated, and very stressful" (Mooney, 1993, p. 44) such a checklist can be for a student. The author stated that the preceptor or skilled nurse knows how to perform tasks presented on a checklist, but when considered from the learners' perspective, the checklist itself becomes a source of anxiety. Mooney conjectured that anxiety then causes decreased attention span, selective listening, narrowed perception, confused thinking, absenteeism, and somatic complaints (Mooney, 1993). While not empirically based, the humorous example gives a different perspective about difficulties students experience when learning/performing a new skill.

Psychomotor skill performance checklists are often a core element of teaching strategy in nursing education. Although checklists are widely used and reported as effective methods of teaching, nursing literature reflects only anecdotal articles on the topic. Research studies would provide needed knowledge with regard to the use of psychomotor skills checklists in nursing education.

Mental Imagery

The use of mental imagery to improve performance on psychomotor skills has been well documented in physical education. In physical education, psychomotor skills are also referred to as kinesthetic skills. When considering the amount of research in physical education addressing the use of mental imagery in performing psychomotor/kinesthetic skills, it is interesting to note that only five research articles were found in the nursing literature.

Eaton and Evans (1986) studied nonspecific imaging practice and how it effects the mental imagery of nursing students; they found that imaging ability of low imagers was enhanced after two practice sessions. Bachman (1990) also explored the usefulness of mental imagery as a technique for practicing psycho-motor skills. Although no significant differences were found in the performance of the study and control groups, participants reported that mental imagery was a useful and interesting learning technique. Bachman (1990) made recommendations for further research to consider subjects' feelings about the psychomotor skill, level of motivation for learning or practicing the skill, and ability to form mental images.

A comparison study was conducted by Smith (1992) using two strategies that consciously link scientific theory with nursing practice. A traditional approach to teaching basic nursing skills was compared with an innovative approach. The traditional mode required the students to complete assigned weekly textbook readings, view films, and study definitions of glossary terms before each laboratory. The innovative strategies were Vee heuristics (a type of mental imagery), which required the student to identify specific concepts, principles, and theories related to basic nursing skills, and concept maps, teaching students how to create schematic drawings of their mental understanding by organizing and linking relevant concepts. Students who were taught basic nursing skills with Vee heuristics and concept maps were better able to identify principles of scientific theory related to basic nursing skills than students in the control group. The author suggested that integration of prior and present knowledge by mental processing reflects meaningful learning; however, research data did not indicate that the treatment group's learning had improved overall skill performance in practice situations.

Doheny (1993) found that high imagers were more proficient at giving an intramuscular injection than low imagers. Doheny (1993) concluded that the ability to use mental practice enhances learning and performance of motor skills. Furthermore, Doheny suggested that research focus on the effectiveness of relaxation as a component of mental practice.

Bucher (1993) explored the interactive effects of imagery skills and various combinations of physical and mental practice on learning a skill. The study found that mental rehearsal in combination with physical practice significantly influenced the learning of a novel psychomotor skill compared to the use of mental rehearsal alone. Bucher concluded that incorporating mental rehearsal as an adjunct to physical practice to facilitate skill acquisition was beneficial.

These studies provide empirical evidence of the effectiveness of mental imagery on learning psychomotor skills. Research should continue to test mental imagery strategies in the development of competence in psychomotor skills. This research has important implications for nursing education. If the positive effect of imagery on learning psychomotor nursing skills is verified, it could become an important strategy in nursing curricula.

Simulation

The simulated clinical laboratory was developed by nursing faculty to be used in the educational setting. Simulations include situations and audiovisual material in conjunction with simulated laboratories. Kolb and Shugart (1984) reported the following activities as simulations: role playing, dramatic representations, simulated patients, selected games, and written or computerized simulations.

A simulation experience was developed by Cowan and Wiens (1986) to examine innovative opportunities for nursing students to refine psychomotor skills before entry into the hospital. To reduce anxiety and increase student competence in communication and psychomotor skills, a mock hospital was set up in the laboratory. This experience was evaluated from student reports. These students perceived that the experience reduced anxiety and provided an opportunity to strengthen psychomotor skills before entering the clinical setting. Nursing faculty reported that students were "more relaxed, moved around the ward more freely and completed nursing care assignments on time" (Cowan & Wiens, 1986, p. 32). While these preliminary findings look promising, the authors cited a need for further research on preclinical practice.

Through simulation, learning situations can be created to provide a context for decision making that is close to reality (McDonald, 1987). McDonald (1987) anecdotally described teaching methods used in a senior clinical course simulation exercise. Focus was placed on nursing interventions in client situations that encompass multiple problems or require rapid decision making, communication, and intervention. Nine educational values were listed as the primary motivation for the development of this experience: variables controlled, learning time maximized, ethical concerns minimized, experimentation and failure allowed, self-evaluation promoted, client feedback elicited, cooperative learning encouraged, and effective decision making promoted. McDonald (1987) recommended that nursing continue to challenge assumptions about the clinical laboratory setting and to develop and study simulation strategies.

Application of critical thinking and decision-making skills are more important than ever given the complexity of technical care involved with client care. This notion led Lowdermilk and Fishel (1991) to study the use of computer simulations in evaluating clinical decision-making skills of 64 senior baccaluareate nursing students enrolled in a clinical course in advanced nursing. The students were randomly assigned to experimental and control groups. All students completed a pretest and posttest that was a computer-assisted instruction clinical simulation specific to the students' clinical placement and a 36-item attitudinal and evaluative questionnaire developed for the study. Although all students demonstrated that significant learning had occurred during the semester, there was no difference between the students who completed the full computer-assisted instruction series and those who did not. Students were found to have positive attitudes toward use of the computer instruction.

The effect of intensive care simulation on anxiety of nursing students in the clinical intensive care unit (ICU) was studied by Erler and Rudman (1993). This study was conducted with junior-level nursing students in a baccalaureate program. The authors found no significant differences in anxiety among students who participated in a simulation and those who did not before attending a clinical experience. Erler and Rudman (1993) concluded that familiarity with psychomotor skills alone is not sufficient to decrease anxiety in the critical care clinical setting.

In a program evaluation of nurse clinicians, an innovative strategy was used to demonstrate skills competence. Simulation exercises using fun and games were created and evaluated by Bradbury-Golas and Carson (1994) in a descriptive study. The authors developed and implemented a nursing skills fair to showcase competence of nursing staff members at skills stations. The stations involved participation by staff members and consisted of skills/equipment not used daily. Nursing participants included approximately 150 registered and practical nurses. The five stations rated most beneficial by the nurses were mechanical ventilation/suctioning, mock code, arterial blood gases, chest tubes, and pediatric IV therapy. The participants evaluated the experience as positive due to the relaxed atmosphere (refreshments and door prizes were provided) and self-guided learning stations. Evaluations included the following suggestions for future fairs: adding several stations (such as specialty beds and traction), holding longer sessions, and implementing the fair three times per year (Bradbury-Golas & Carson, 1994). Due to reported success of the nursing skills fair, the techniques should be explored for use in the nursing skills laboratory with beginning students.

White (1995) compared the use of problem solving with computer simulations and actual patients. A quasi-experimental design was developed, and criterion validity of the simulations was established. 16 nursing students were asked to evaluate their perceptions of the similarity between caring for simulated and actual patients. The study reported that 75% thought the simulations were similar or very similar to actual clinical encounters. Additionally, the author reported that use of computer-based patient simulations with interactive videotape allows teaching not possible with computer-based patient simulations without video. Interactive video allows students to "see" the patient they are interviewing and to "examine" the patient rather than having the examination findings described by the software developer (White, 1995). It was further suggested that videotape allows students to integrate laboratory and other diagnostic findings into the care of the computer-simulated patient. The study was limited by sample size to 16 nursing students.

Simulations will continue to play an integral role in developing psychomotor nursing skills and incorporating them into the greater context of nursing care. This method of teaching offers a safe means for the student to practice skills before entering the actual patient setting, makes efficient use of time and resources, and allows the student to make decisions about client care in the laboratory setting. The changing health care environment will likely increase the demand for teaching by simulation exercises, thus increasing the demand for research to guide teaching practice.

Multimedia

Few studies are available on teaching psychomotor skills with various aspects of multimedia and the clinical setting. Oermann (1990) found a large body of research in nursing education on the effectiveness of multimedia; however, few studies focused on using media (videotape and computer-assisted instruction) for clinical teaching. Following a review of research on multimedia, Oermann (1990) concluded that media were as effective as other teaching methods in helping students acquire knowledge relevant to clinical practice and develop beginning practice skills. The author found that in some of the research comparing the effectiveness of media to lecture, clinical performance was included as a dependent variable. The findings indicated that media were at least as effective as lecture and lecture-discussion in improving clinical performance.

A few studies are available that specifically focus on teaching psychomotor skills with varying media and in various settings. Baldwin, Hill, and Hanson (1991) compared two teaching strategies—textbook assignment and videotaping with no faculty assistance, and textbook assignment and videotaping with faculty guidance—to determine the effect on proficiency at measuring blood pressure. Students were randomly assigned to one of these groups, and a significant difference was found between groups. These authors found that while videotaping may be used for learning skills, faculty contact during the instruction was important. It was suggested that further research examine student/faculty contact time and its effects on psychomotor performance outcomes.

Another area that needs further research is the interaction of different learner characteristics and use of multimedia and the effect of these on learning outcomes. Following a review of literature, Thompson and Crutchlow (1993) suggested that using various media in the teaching setting makes use of different strengths and develops different skills. The types of media suggested to develop these strengths and skills were: reading, viewing films, using computer-assisted instruction, engaging in role play, conducting nursing rounds, and participating in case discussion.

McDonald (1987) described the use of video and telephone role play in which client situations were designed and simulated. This study was developed by nursing faculty as a cost-saving strategy in response to pressures from the affiliated hospital to decrease the number of nursing students in the emergency department. The study was reported as effective in monitoring students' ability to teach clients. McDonald (1987) found that while educational values were realized, clinical simulation has some limitations, including time/preparation, content development, availability of equipment, and student anxiety about role playing. The author recommended that we continue to challenge our assumptions about the clinical laboratory setting and to study simulation strategies in an atmosphere of cost containment.

Love, McAdams, Patton, Rankin, and Roberts (1989) conducted a randomized control trial to compare the effectiveness of teaching psychomotor skills in a structured laboratory setting with self-directed, self-taught modules. The authors obtained a sample of 77 sophomore baccalaureate nursing students. The study found no difference between the psychomotor skill performance of students who learn in a self-directed manner and those taught in a structured clinical laboratory. Therefore, the authors concluded that teaching psychomotor skills in a self-directed learning approach may be as effective as

time application of the skill in a patient situation. The author suggested that the decline in anxiety after the laboratory class indicates that the students benefitted from this instructional experience. Overall, the findings supported preclinical skill evaluation as an effective strategy for reducing anxiety related to initial transfer of skill learning from a laboratory to a clinical setting and enhancing self-confidence. The study was limited to beginning students and one complex skill. Additional investigation was recommended to determine the effectiveness of preclinical skill evaluation with advanced students and other skills of varying complexity. Based upon these findings, the author suggested further investigation on the effect of review/rehearsal on performance of skills.

Gomez and Gomez (1987) studied learning of psychomotor skills in a laboratory versus patient care setting. Open and closed motor skills theory was used to categorize skills according to the environmental context in which the skills were performed. A closed psychomotor skill was defined as performance in stable and stationary environments, and an open psychomotor skill was defined as performance in dynamic environments (Gomez & Gomez, 1987).

Gomez and Gomez (1987) examined strategies used to teach psychomotor skills in nursing. The authors found eight studies investigating the presentation of information concerning the skill to be learned and two studies that investigated the use of videotape for student feedback. In reviewing the literature, Gomez and Gomez (1987) found no study in nursing education investigating practice conditions when learning a nursing psychomotor skill. Gomez and Gomez (1987) designed a study to investigate practice conditions when learning a psychomotor skill in a bachelor's degree program in nursing. The subjects consisted of 63 students in two upper division programs enrolled in first-level nursing courses. Practice on a postpartum gynecological floor in a general hospital was compared to practice in the college laboratory. Skill attainment was evaluated in a nursing home using performance criteria. The skill investigated was measuring blood pressure (an open psychomotor skill). The subjects were randomly assigned to one of two groups for practice: patient care setting or college laboratory. The college laboratory group served as the control group. The most significant finding of the study was that the group who practiced taking blood pressure in the patient care setting scored higher on a checklist on a competency checklist than the group who practiced in the college setting. There was no evidence of any difference between the two practice groups (evaluators and subjects) when measuring systolic and diastolic readings (right and left arms). The patient care setting group demonstrated greater confidence in taking blood pressure compared to the college laboratory group. One explanation for the findings may have been the large differences between practice and evaluation settings and type of clients (postpartum in-patient and elderly nursing home). The authors recommended seeking alternatives to traditional patient care settings if these sites become less readily available. Suggested alternative settings were clinics, day care centers for children, units for the chronically ill, rehabilitation centers, elderly centers, and screening centers.

Use of technological equipment in the clinical setting was examined by Pelletier (1995), who studied how diploma-prepared registered nurses from tertiary institutions perceived their ability to handle technical equipment in the workplace. A questionnaire was developed to determine frequency of use of specified clinical equipment and graduates' degree of comfort in handling this equipment during their educational program and in the workplace as registered nurses. The graduates' belief in the need for competency in using each item prior to graduation and factors that influenced this belief were also determined. Commonly used items of clinical equipment specified were glucometers, nasogastric pumps, infusion control devices, electronic syphgmomanometers, cardiac monitors, electronic thermometers, 12-lead electrocardiographs, lifting devices, and suction pumps. The questionnaire was completed by 245 diploma registered nurses. The most frequently used equipment included the glucose-measuring devices, intravenous infusion devices, and nasogastric pumps for enteral feeding, which the authors suggested reflects the trend toward a greater number of acutely ill patients. The authors did not find a significant relationship between frequently used items of clinical equipment and whether the item caused the nurse concern in practice. Additionally, findings did not support a significant relationship between the frequent use of an item and whether participants believed that competence with the item should be acquired prior to graduation. The study found that graduates expressed a need for a level of competence with specific equipment prior to entry into the workforce. Thus, the authors suggested that nurse educators need to consider how competency can be achieved more effectively either in the classroom or through more effective utilization of the clinical practice experience.

The findings of these studies have implications for teaching nursing students in both the classroom and clinical setting. Based on these findings it is important not to assume that the most frequently used items should be the main focus in the teaching program. As mentioned previously, further investigation is warranted with teaching psychomotor nursing skills in the educational program and regarding the setting in which specific skills are best learned.

LEARNER VARIABLES

Learner variables have been addressed throughout the literature as learning styles and demographic characteristics (age, gender, culture). Throughout general educational literature, literally hundreds of studies can be found addressing learning styles as a learner variable. However, only two evidence-based studies were found in nursing literature that related specifically to learning psychomotor skills in nursing, and only one critical review of literature. This is surprising, given the general use of student demographic characteristics to predict success in nursing programs and on the National Council Licensure Examination (NCLEX). Learning style has received much attention because of its potential to explain variations in student outcomes, given the same educational experience. Meta-analysis of general education research on learning styles concludes that learning style matched with teaching style does not make a difference in outcome.

Nursing literature contains two evidence-based articles related to learning styles as a learner variable. Goldsmith (1984) supported the notion that the teaching style used can affect student learning. The author reported that limited information is available to assist faculty in selecting and designing audiovisual media to maximize learning for individuals with differing abilities. Goldsmith (1984) found a variety of methodological and theoretical problems in previous research: (a) The design of experiments focused on finding the best medium for instruction rather than determining how a medium effects learning; (b) studies failed to consider interactions between media variables and learning tasks; (c) there was poor conceptualization of media variables when comparing gross physical characteristics of media (such as television versus face-to-face lecture); and (d) the unique presentation attributes of media were not compared (such as the ability to show an object in motion versus the ability to show only a static picture of the object). Due to these limitations in prior research, Goldsmith (1984) designed a study to investigate the interactions between three learner aptitudes and two treatment variables associated with learning a psychomotor nursing skill. Two personality variables (state anxiety and trait anxiety) and one cognitive-style variable (field orientation) were measured. The treatment variables were media presentation (videotape and slide-tape) and learning condition (practice on a mannequin versus practice on a real person playing the part of a patient). The task studied was changing of a sterile dressing on an abdominal wound with a penrose drain. The research design was a 2 × 2 factorial design with two levels of media treatment and two levels of learning condition. The study failed to find significant media–learner relationships with respect to psychomotor learning; however, the author reported that the aptitude-by-treatment interaction design may be a useful approach for future investigations involving instructional media. The study found that trait anxiety, state anxiety, and field orientation are not critical individual difference variables affecting the psychomotor learning from a videotape or slidetape program. Goldsmith (1984) suggested that future research examine the effect of the instructional strategy over a longer period of time, since this study evaluated the effect of the aptitude measures only in an immediate posttest of the learning. In addition, it was suggested that further research address the limited sample size of 55 subjects.

In the study conducted by Lowdermilk and Fishel (1991), Kolb's Learning Style Inventory was given to 64 senior baccalaureate nursing students enrolled in a clinical course in advanced nursing. The questionnaire was included to determine if there was a relationship between student learning style preference and computer-assisted instruction scores. It was found that success on the computer-assisted instruction was independent of learning style.

Thompson and Crutchlow (1993) conducted a critical review of the education and nursing literature regarding learning styles and found that the concept of learning styles and its relationship to academic achievement had been extensively researched. The authors found that generally, the literature suggests that the planning of teaching strategies be guided by an assessment of students' learning styles. In addition, some writers advocated matching students' learning style with teaching style to optimize learning. Although Thompson and Crutchlow (1993) found much written about the implications of learning styles on the teaching/learning process, they suggested that these implications be used with caution. The suggested validity of findings was jeopardized by several methodological deficiencies including lack of a clear and consistent definition of learning styles, the use of small study samples, and inadequate research designs. Thus, there was much inconsistency in the findings of studies reviewed by these authors. Two important factors found missing in much of the literature reviewed by Thompson and Crutchlow (1993) were the influence of the environment on learning and the influence of cultural background. The review found that research on learning/cognitive style produced mixed results. No conclusive evidence was found that style affects the learning process. Consequently, it was suggested that nurse educators critically review research findings before applying them to the educational setting. Furthermore, the authors suggested that nursing is a dynamic profession and demands that students be taught in flexible ways in order to appropriately apply knowledge in different settings as well as with different individuals.

The amount of knowledge about learner variables in the educational literature, with respect to the limited information found in the nursing literature, provides a springboard from which to develop research. The problems with methodology, sample size, and research design need to be addressed in future research. With the variety of individuals encountered in the educational setting, it is important to have a knowledge base and framework from which to make decisions that provide the most effective teaching/learning environment for psychomotor nursing skills acquisition.

CONCLUSIONS

Implications for Nursing Education

While nursing is beginning to document evidence from research and the implications for teaching psychomotor nursing skills, more investigation is needed in this area. Until this research is conducted and findings are reported, it is recommended that teaching decisions be based on teaching/learning principles. As these studies emerge, their results should be implemented where appropriate. Nurse educators must incorporate change and adaptability into the learning laboratory, to prepare nursing students who are marketable for the twenty-first century.

Need for Further Research

Changes in the health care setting and delivery methods have presented faculty with challenges for creating learning experiences. This came about when nursing education moved from the practice setting into formal education, health care reform moved patients quickly from acute care to home care, emphasis was placed on health promotion and health care costs, and rapid changes developed in technology (both in the clinical setting and in the laboratory). To address these changes, nursing faculty developed simulated experiences to teach psychomotor skills in the learning resource center. These dynamic processes continue to shape and mold the methods by which these skills are being taught. This review of literature provides an overview of knowledge about teaching psychomotor skills within nursing education.

The limited number of research studies found in this review, along with mixed findings, warrants further investigation of the nursing laboratory and psychomotor skills. Research is needed on psychomotor nursing skills and teaching methods that most effectively encourage development of these kinesthetic skills among learners. The use of multimedia and the relationship of multimedia to skill performance needs to be explored. Developing valid and reliable measures of teaching psychomotor skills remains an important goal. Testing is warranted with large samples, varying levels of nursing students, different types of nursing programs, multiple settings, and nurse clinicians. Further research should examine the interaction of different learner characteristics and the effect of these on learning. As seen in other nursing research, there is lack of replication in the setting of the original research and with different populations, sample size is limited, and validity and reliability of measurement data need to be established.

REFERENCES

Alavi, C., Loh, S. H., & Reilly, D. (1991). Reality basis for teaching psychomotor skills in a tertiary nursing curriculum. *Journal of Advanced Nursing, 16*(8) 957–965.

Anderson, B., Conklin, D., Watson, L., Hirst, S., & Hoffman, J. (1985). Psychomotor skills for baccalaureates. *The Australian Nurses Journal, 15*(3), 40–43.

Bachman, K. (1990). Using mental imagery to practice a specific psychomotor skill. *Journal of Continuing Education in Nursing, 21*(3), 125–128.

Baldwin, D., Hill, P., & Hanson, G. (1991). Performance of psychomotor skills: A comparison of two teaching strategies. *Journal of Nursing Education, 30*(8), 367–370.

Bell, M. (1991). Learning a complex nursing skill: Student anxiety and the effect of preclinical skill evaluation. *Journal of Nursing Education, 30*(5), 222–226.

Benner, P. (1984). *From novice to expert.* Menlo Park, CA: Addison-Wesley.

Bevis, E. O., & Clayton, G. (1988). Needed: A new curriculum development design. *Nurse Educator, 13*(4), 14–18.

Bjork, I. T. (1995). Neglected conflicts in the discipline of nursing: Perceptions of the importance and value of practical skill. *Journal of Advanced Nursing, 22*(1), 6–12.

Bolton, J. G. (1984). Educating professional nurses for clinical practice. *Nursing and Health Care, 5*(7), 385–389.

Bradbury-Golas, K., & Carson, L. (1994). Nursing skills fair: Gaining knowledge with fun and games. *Journal of Continuing Education in Nursing,* 25(1), 32–34.

Brigham, C. J., Foster, S. L., & Hodson, K. E. (1991). A participatory learning module: Asepsis and universal precautions. *Nurse Educator, 16*(1), 22–25.

Bucher, L. (1993). The effects of imagery abilities and mental rehearsal on learning a nursing skill evaluation. *Journal of Nursing Education, 32*(7), 318–324.

Corcoran, S. (1977). Should a service setting be used as a learning laboratory? *Nursing Outlook, 25*(12) 771–776.

Cowan, D., & Wiens, V. (1986). Mock hospital: A preclinical laboratory experience. *Nurse Educator, 11*(5), 30–32.

Dave, R. H. (1970). *Psychomotor levels in developing and writing behavioural objectives.* Tucson, AZ. Educational Innovators Press.

de Tornyay, R., & Thompson, M. A. (1987). *Strategies for teaching nursing* (3rd ed.). New York: Wiley.

del Bueno, D., Weeks, L., & Brown-Stewart, P. (1987). Clinical assessment centers: A cost-effective alternative for competency development. *Nursing Economics, 5*(1), 21–26.

Doheny, M. (1993). Mental practice: An alternative approach to teaching motor skills. *Journal of Nursing Education, 32*(6), 260–264.

Dreyfus, S. E., & Dreyfus, H. L. (1980). *A five-stage model of the mental activities involved in directed skill acquisition.* Unpublished manuscript, University of California at Berkeley.

Eaton, S. L., & Evans, S. B. (1986). The effect of nonspecific imaging practice on the mental imagery ability of nursing students acquisition of psychomotor skills. *Journal of Nursing Education, 25*(5), 193–196.

Elliott, R., Jillings, C., & Thorne, S. (1982). Psychomotor skill acquisition in nursing students in Canada and the U.S. *Canadian Nurse, 78*(3), 25–27.

Erler, C. J., & Rudman, S. D. (1993). Effect of intensive care simulation on anxiety of nursing students in the clinical ICU. *Heart and Lung: Journal of Critical Care, 22*(3), 259–265.

Field, W. E., Gallman, L., Nicholson, R., & Dreher, M. (1984). Clinical competencies of baccalaureate students. *Journal of Nursing Education, 23*(7), 284–293.

Garcia, C. B. (1988). *A comparison of head nurses' expectations for the psychomotor skill competencies of entry level professional nurses with the expectations of nursing instructors for their graduates from associate degree, diploma, and baccalaureate degree nursing programs.* Unpublished manuscript, Boston College.

Goldsmith, J. W. (1984). Effect of learner variables, media attributes, and practice condition on psychomotor task performance. *Western Journal of Nursing Research, 6*(2), 229–240.

Gomez, G. E., & Gomez, E. A. (1987). Learning of psychomotor skills: Laboratory versus patient care setting. *Journal of Nursing Education, 26*(1), 20–24.

Gudmundsen, A. (1975). Teaching psychomotor skills. *Journal of Nursing Education, 14*(1), 23–27.

Hallal, J. C. & Welsh, M. D. (1984). Using the competency laboratory to learn psychomotor skills. *Nurse Educator, 9*(1), 34–38.

Hodson, K.E., Brigham, C., Hanson, A., & Armstrong, K. (1988). Multimedia simulation of a clinical day. *Nurse Educator, 13*(1), 10–13.

Hodson, K. E., Manis, J., Thayer, M., Webb, S., Hunnicutt, C., & Hoogenboom, A. (1988). Computerized management program for the skills laboratory of a school of nursing. *Computers in Nursing, 6*(5), 215–221.

Kieffer, J. F. (1984). Teaching technical skills for competency. *Journal of Nursing Education, 23*(5), 198–203.

Kolb, S. E., & Shugart, E. B. (1984). Evaluation: Is simulation the answer? *Journal of Nursing Education, 23*(2), 84–86.

Love, B., McAdams, C., Patton, D. M., Rankin, E. J., & Roberts, J. (1989). Teaching psychomotor skills in nursing: A randomized control trial. *Journal of Advanced Nursing, 14,* 970–975.

Lowdermilk, D., & Fishel, A. H. (1991). Computer simulations as a measure of nursing students' decision-making skills. *Journal of Nursing Education, 30,* 34–39.

McCaffrey, C. (1978). Performance checklists: An effective method of teaching, learning, and evaluating. *Nurse Educator, 3,* 11–13.

McDonald, G. F. (1987). The simulated clinical laboratory, *Nursing Outlook, 35*(6), 290–292.

Miller, K. H. (1989). *A comparison of the perceptions of nursing faculty and nursing service personnel on psychomotor competencies for graduate baccalaureate nurses.* Unpublished manuscript, Boston University.

Mooney, N. (1993). Juggling performance checklist . . . teaching psychomotor skills to nurses. *Journal of Continuing Education in Nursing, 24*(1), 43–44.

Oermann, M. (1990). Psychomotor skill development. *Journal of Continuing Education in Nursing, 21*(5), 202–204.

Pelletier, D. (1995). Diploma-prepared nurses' use of technological equipment in clinical practice. *Journal of Advanced Nursing, 21*(1), 6–14.

Richardson, A. (1969). *Mental imagery.* New York: Springer.

Smith, B. E. (1992). Linking theory and practice in teaching basic nursing skills. *Journal of Nursing Education, 32,* 16–23.

Stern, S. B. (1988). Are we preparing baccalaureate students for practice? *Nurse Educator, 13*(4), 3–4.

Studdy, S. J., Nicol, M. J., & Fox-Hiley, A. (1994). Teaching and learning clinical skills: Part 2. Development of a teaching model and schedule of skills development. *Nurse Education Today, 14*(3), 186–193.

Sweeney, M. A., Hedstrom, B., & O'Malley, M. (1982). Process evaluation: A second look at psychomotor skills. *Journal of Nursing Education, 21*(2), 4–16.

Sweeney, M. A., & Regan, A. (1982). Educators, employees, and new graduates define essential skills for baccalaureate graduates. *The Journal of Nursing Administration, 12,* 36–42.

Thompson, C., & Crutchlow, E. (1993). Learning style research: A critical review of the literature and implications for nursing education. *Journal of Professional Nursing, 9*(1), 34–40.

Urick, J., & Bond, E. (1994). Self-instructional laboratories revisited by high technology. *Computers in Nursing, 12*(1), 5–6.

White, J. E., (1995). Using interactive video to add physical assessment data to computer-based patient simulations in nursing. *Computers in Nursing, 13*(5), 233–235.

Wooley, A. (1977). The long and tortured history of clinical evaluation. *Nursing Outlook, 25*(5), 308–315.

Chapter 4

Academic Dishonesty: Addressing the Problems of Cheating, Plagiarism, and Professional Misconduct

MARTHA J. BRADSHAW, RN, PHD
ARLENE LOWENSTEIN, RN, PHD

INTRODUCTION

Academic dishonesty, in the forms of cheating on tests and assignments, plagiarism, and lying, has been a long-standing problem in higher education (Baird, 1980; Davis & Ludvigson, 1995; Roth & McCabe, 1995; Westerman, Grandy, Lupo, & Tamisiea, 1996). Unfortunately, the incidence of academic dishonesty is increasing (Anderson & Obenshain, 1994; McCabe & Trevino, 1996). In professional education, this problem is especially disconcerting because of the link between academic and professional ethics. In health care professions, such as nursing, altruism, service, and standards of professional ethical conduct are central to maintaining the integrity of the profession. Neophyte professionals are guided by faculty in developing a code of ethics and understanding professional standards. Academic as well as professional dishonesty cannot coexist with these standards. Therefore, faculty are challenged not only to instruct students in professional codes but also to be alert to lapses in ethical conduct and to intervene effectively in such situations.

Because of the serious consequences of dishonest behavior, contributing factors must be identified and modified, and faculty must be equipped with the means to counsel, remediate, or dismiss students. In order to achieve these means, faculty must understand academic dishonesty and faculty–student interaction in the process. This chapter reviews research and related literature regarding academic dishonesty in higher education, with an emphasis on professional students. A model of factors contributing to academic dishonesty is presented, along with recommendations for interventions. Additionally, the chapter discusses legal implications for faculty and educational programs that come from litigation cases in situations of academic dishonesty.

To facilitate database searches needed for this review, the terms pertinent to the concept of academic dishonesty were identified. English dictionaries and thesauruses were consulted to identify words synonymous with academic dishonesty. Words selected as most appropriate for this review are cheating, plagiarism, and lying. The phrase *unethical professional behavior* was also used as a keyword relevant to academic dishonesty in nursing education. To further organize and present this review, definitions of the keywords were developed, based upon a consensus of their usage in the publications reviewed.

Cheating is defined as any intentional, deceitful, or dishonest behavior that is considered inappropriate or unethical (Barnett & Dalton, 1981). These behaviors include providing or receiving unauthorized information on examinations, falsifying information or submitting written information without accurately documenting sources, and generally claiming any submitted assignment as one's own when it is not. *Plagiarism* is the appropriation or falsification of formal work, usually in writing. Plagiarism can range from poor paraphrasing to intentional verbatim copying that does not credit the original source (Hawley, 1984). Plagiarism can be a complex problem due to the difficulty of proving intent to falsify versus ignorance over citation methods (Bradshaw & Lowenstein, 1990). Plagiarism is also problematic because it raises questions regarding violation of copyright law (Mawdsley, 1985). *Lying* has been defined as conscious awareness of a falsity with the intent to deceive (Ford, King, & Hollender, 1988) *Unethical professional behavior* in health care settings consists of acts that might compromise patient care (Vargo, 1991). Unethical professional behaviors can take place in either class or clinical practice settings and have been defined as a broad range of actions generally considered by educators as being dishonest or fraudulent (Hilbert, 1985).

Electronic database searches were conducted of Cumulative Index to Nursing and Allied Health Literature (CINAHL), Medline, ERIC, Psychological Abstracts, Dissertation Abstracts, and Education Abstracts for the years 1986 through 1996. To facilitate identification and selection of relevant articles, the limiting terms *college* and *faculty* were used. Additionally, the tables of contents for *Nurse Educator* and *Journal of Nursing Education* from 1985 to 1996 were examined to identify pertinent publications. To be suitable for this review, the following criteria must be met: (a) article must be English language and must address students or faculty in higher education settings, in either undergraduate, graduate, or professional programs; (b) article must be either a research report regarding an aspect of academic dishonesty or a theory-based publication that either describes or explains academic dishonesty or offers recommendations; (c) research articles must report the design, sample, method of data collection and analysis, and results.

A total of 164 articles that met at least one of the criteria were identified. Of these articles, 22 met all three criteria established for this chapter and therefore are reviewed in depth. Articles that met only one or two of the criteria were included in the chapter to provide additional background on academic dishonesty. Additionally, research and related articles from 1964 through 1985 were selected as relevant when cited in studies as key support to later work. An unpublished study by one of the chapter authors is included for further evidence.

Of the 22 studies reviewed, three of the articles reported research that explored theory development or contributed to a theoretical model of academic dishonesty. One study was a review of honor code policies. The remaining articles reported on incidences of academic dishonesty or opinions by students or faculty. The most common research method used in the reviewed studies was quantitative, and the most frequent design was descriptive, either by questionnaire or by rating scale ($N = 18$). One study had a *post hoc* comparative design. Three studies used qualitative methodology, employing interview ($N = 2$) and observation ($N = 1$) designs. To select subjects, all studies used convenience samples. In the review section of this chapter, individual studies will be identified that used selective groups versus those that used an entire student population from one or more schools.

Nine studies focused on undergraduate students in general programs, three investigated professional undergraduate nursing students, two studied graduate students in nonprofessional programs, and four examined graduate professional students in either medical or dental school. Four studies did not identify the academic level of the subjects, but referred to them as "college students" or just "students." Two studies compared findings in undergraduate students to findings in graduate students, and one of these studies investigated students in allied health programs. Of all the research studies, three involved students and faculty, and two were restricted to faculty as subjects. Seventeen of the research studies investigated cheating, lying, and plagiarism in some combination. The one study that used subject observation examined cheating situations exclusively. An additional four studies examined unprofessional or unethical clinical behaviors along with cheating, lying, or plagiarism. One study investigated unethical behaviors, accompanied by cheating or lying, in master's of business administration (MBA) students.

REVIEW OF LITERATURE

Academic dishonesty, causative or circumstantial factors, and disciplinary measures have been described adequately in general higher education literature. Some studies have been conducted with students in health professions, but little literature is focused specifically on nursing students. An overview of academic dishonesty is called for because the numerous issues in this higher education problem are directly related to nursing education, predominantly with undergraduate students. Therefore, the review of research literature will present those studies available, emphasizing findings that are applicable to nursing students. This review focuses on three perspectives of academic dishonesty. One perspective, found in the section on causative or contributing factors, looks at the psychological underpinnings that preclude various dishonest behaviors. These underpinnings are either long-standing unethical, dishonest, or deceitful behaviors in the student, selected defense mechanisms that make academic dishonesty acceptable to the individual, or conscious, short-term behaviors that precede an episode of spontaneous cheating. The second perspective focuses on a profile of students who engage in academic dishonesty. Demographic data that emerged from the studies reviewed present a student profile that can enable faculty to better understand and address academic dishonesty in students. The third perspective involves the attitudes toward academic dishonesty held by both students and college faculty. This section includes studies that focused on attitudes held by either students or faculty, as well as some studies that compared views on the problem between the two groups.

In addition to reviewing and discussing the research and related literature, this chapter will critique individual studies and summarize findings as they relate to nursing education. Specific recommendations for faculty who must address academic dishonesty are part of the section on implications for nursing education.

Causative or Contributing Factors

Based on reviewed literature, Bradshaw and Lowenstein (1990) developed a model of factors contributing to academic dishonesty (Figure 4–1). They

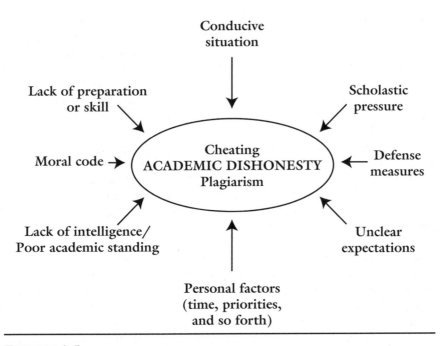

FIGURE 4-1.
Factors Contributing to Academic Dishonesty.
Bradshaw, M. J., & Lowenstein, A. (1990). Perspectives on academic
dishonesty. **Nurse Educator, 15(5), 10–15. Reprinted by permission.**

noted that a variety of factors which contribute to academic dishonesty operate singularly or simultaneously within the student. Baird (1980) characterized cheating by college students as either a long-standing, complex problem or a one-time instance occurring as a result of lack of study time, other priorities, or low interest in the course or exam. Underlying personal attributes also contribute to dishonest behaviors. Baumeister and Scher (1988) described the typical cheater, who prefers the immediate short-term benefit derived from cheating, as also being an individual who exercises poor judgment in other areas of life. Hetherington and Feldman (1964) explained that individuals who tend to cheat have a personally identified need to cheat as well as personality characteristics that enable cheating. A conducive situation is the remaining variable needed to bring about an incidence of cheating , but cheating still calls for an unethical or risk-taking individual (Uhlig & Howes, 1967). Thus, the reasons why students cheat have been attributed to short-term, situational factors (personal priorities, environment) as well as long-standing psychological issues. This model and the related research have been supported by more recent studies.

In a seminal study by Baird (1980), subjects reported that cheating in college was not unusual. The subjects, college undergraduate students ($N = 200$), cited the primary reasons for cheating as desire for good grades, inadequate time for studying, and heavy workload. More simplistically put, students cheat to avoid failing a class (Nuss, 1984) or to get a higher course grade (Davis & Ludvigson, 1995). In addition to these reasons, Genereux and McLeod (1995) cited financial support linked with academic success as a reason for cheating. Barnett and Dalton (1981) believe that pressure and competition for grades is "unquestionably the single most important cause of academic dishonesty" (p. 549).

Many incidences of cheating are the result of opportunistic behaviors. That is, when circumstances are conducive to cheating, such as with poor proctoring or a close seating arrangement, students will take advantage of the situation; importance of the test also influences whether students cheat. These findings have been supported in a small study of 46 students in college English and psychology classes (Uhlig & Howes, 1967), a study of 365 college students in various programs (Genereux & McLeod, 1995), a study of 2,459 medical students (Baldwin, Daugherty, Rowley, & Schwarz, 1996), and an overview of studies by (Baird, 1980). Conversely, high instructor vigilance, interest in the students, and clarity of disciplinary ramifications related to academic dishonesty are deterrents to cheating (Davis & Ludvigson, 1995; Genereux & McLeod, 1995).

A conducive situation may be especially appealing to students who take risks in other aspects of their lives. Baumeister and Scher (1988) noted risk-taking behavior in some individuals who prefer the short-term benefit, for example, a good course grade, over a long-term, perhaps unforeseen cost such as poor clinical judgment. The student, thus, is able to justify dishonest behavior for the immediate gain.

Hetherington and Feldman (1964) identified four types of cheating behaviors:

Independent opportunistic—cheating is impulsive and unplanned.

Independent planned—cheating evolves out of planning and pretest activity.

Social active and *social passive*—two or more people are involved, with cheating instigated by one individual and the others allowing it to occur.

In a study with 78 undergraduate students in a child psychology course, the investigators developed actual situations conducive to cheating. 59% of the subjects seized the opportunity to cheat, either by using crib notes, peeking at the textbook, or copying from others. In analyzing the incidences of cheating with demographic information and results of personality tests, Hetherington and Feldman found that cheating was more common in males and/or first-born subjects and in subjects who were more passive-dependent. These subjects put little effort into either intellectual development or social relationships. Additionally, the cheaters in this study, as in other studies, had lower grades and were more likely to use repressive defense mechanisms. Socially passive cheaters were identified as subjects who were concerned with sustaining relationships and cheated to be accepted. Opportunistic cheaters were more impulsive, poorly socialized, and unconventional. The findings in this study indicate that seizing an opportunity to cheat is different from the thought processes accompanying planned cheating behaviors, such as plagiarism. According to Hetherington and Feldman, students who will use an opportunity to cheat on an examination will not purposely plagiarize, and students who plagiarize do so because it provides a controlled, planned vehicle for improving a grade.

Dishonest behaviors that are intentional and planned are part of a psychic mechanism that may include longevity, self-protection, and ethical disregard. Elements associated with lying and planned cheating behaviors include preconceived purpose, consciousness of falsity, and conscious intent to deceive (Ford et al., 1988). A personality structure that includes incorporating dishonest behavior into personal schemata seems to result in a repeat or chronic cheater. A study by Baldwin et al. (1996) of medical students revealed that previous cheating episodes are the best predictors of cheating in medical school, and that the students reporting such acts perceived that cheating was impossible to eliminate.

In some studies (Bradshaw, 1989; Genereux & McLeod, 1995), reasons for cheating were attributional. The students said the subject matter was of low importance/low interest, the course was too difficult or too time consuming, classmates were also cheating, or the instructor either was a poor teacher or did not care about them as students and did not care whether they cheated. Attributional theory, whether conscious or subconscious, enables the individual to develop a personally justifiable reason for engaging in unethical behavior.

A similar defense mechanism employed by students engaging in academic dishonesty is neutralization or rationalization. This mechanism can be used at any time during the commission of a dishonest act to deflect negative attributes, such as disapproval, away from oneself and others. In doing so, individuals free themselves from the moral obligation to uphold the law and eliminate any sense of guilt (Haines, Diekhoff, LaBeff, & Clark, 1986). Not surprisingly, in studying 380 undergraduate students, Haines et al. (1986) found higher levels of neutralization among students who also admitted to having cheated while in college. Examples of neutralizing statements used by this group were, "His cheating isn't hurting anyone" and "The people sitting around him made no attempt to cover their papers." These investigators associated neutralization with low moral development and found such neutralizing acts occurring in students who were younger, more dependent upon parents for financial support, and less committed to their academic work (e.g., lower grade point averages [GPAs], more extracurricular activities).

Payne and Nantz (1994) agreed that cheating is strongly associated with attribution, rationalization, excuses, and other form of self-preservation. They did not limit academic dishonesty to these psychic mechanisms but believed that misconduct is a "social reality" that is part of the student culture. This could explain why dishonest behavior, especially cheating, is both widespread and accepted. In a qualitative study with 41 upper division undergraduates, Payne and Nantz (1994) found that students were able to categorize and explain their reasons for cheating through various metaphors. Personal values ("I see no reason why I should not do it"), organization ("The university treats me unfairly"), and economics ("It would save money or make money for me") are three of the 14 categories that emerged from this study. Metaphors to account for cheating included "a game, " "an addiction, " and a "team effort."

Self-concept and outside influences have a part in commission of a dishonest act. Anderson and Obenshain (1994) described cheaters as having lower grade point averages and being less self-sufficient, more extroverted, and more ambitious. However, Roig and Neaman (1994) linked alienation with low GPA and tendency toward cheating. A possible explanation is that an extroverted, ambitious student may cheat in order to feel less alienated.

These psychic mechanisms, at work simultaneously with optimal academic circumstances, provide a means for cheating or plagiarism and thus explain Bradshaw and Lowenstein's (1990) model of academic dishonesty. Regardless of the circumstances, the fact that students engage in dishonest behavior indicates a lapse in moral judgment. This and related psychological issues are of central concern to educators in professional programs (Ozar, 1991). Students who become accustomed to cheating, lying, and engaging in other dishonest acts will view them as normal and will carry the behaviors to other settings, such as patient care.

Academic Dishonesty: Demographics, Frequency, and Types of Incidences

Undergraduate Students. Incidences of academic dishonesty, especially cheating, have been documented by educational researchers for over 50 years (Baird, 1980). A study by McCabe and Trevino (1996) revealed dramatic increases in dishonest behaviors from 1963 to 1993. Incidences of copying from another student rose from 26% to 52%, and plagiarism showed a small rise from 49% to 54%. Unapproved collaboration on assignments increased noticeably from 11% to 49%. One interesting drop is that today's students seem less inclined to turn in work that has been done by another: The authors reported that submission of work done by another occurred in 19% of subjects studied in 1963 and only 14% of subjects studied in 1993 (McCabe & Trevino, 1996).

Reports vary on what seems to be the most common types of academic dishonesty. Cheating, in the form of giving and receiving exam answers either before or during the test, was the most frequent transgression found by Genereux and McLeod (1995), and plagiarism was the most common in a study by Falleur (1990). Hawley (1984) found acts of plagiarism to occur more often in students who had lower GPAs.

Demographic characteristics have been linked with unethical or dishonest behaviors in educational settings. Frequency of participating in cheating seems to decrease in upper division students (juniors and seniors); that is, the longer students are in college, the less they cheat (Baird, 1980). Davis and Ludvigson (1995) determined that students who cheated in high school continued to do so with their undergraduate, lower division college work. Haines and colleagues (1986) cited immaturity, as a function of age, as a correlate to cheating. When considering reasons why students cheat, such as to get the grade they want, especially to pass the course, it seems logical that the more successful the student is academically, the less he or she needs to cheat. This, of course, could be attributed to a rise in self-esteem following academic success, or the fact that numbers of students who cheat diminish as they are caught, drop out, or fail out of school.

Cheating has been found to occur more frequently among male students in general populations of undergraduate students (Davis & Ludvigson, 1995; Falleur, 1990; Genereux & McLeod, 1995). This finding has not been supported in nursing students (Hilbert, 1985, 1987), which may be a function of a primarily female student population. Hilbert (1985) also reported that many of the males in her first study were married and slightly older than the majority of the female subjects. No studies were found that addressed academic dishonesty in ethnic groups. Only two of the studies reviewed mentioned ethnic groups in the demographic data; in these reports, ethnicity was not found to be significant and no conclusions based upon ethnic groups were derived (Hilbert, 1987; McCabe & Bowers, 1994).

Graduate Students. Academic dishonesty in graduate students has received little attention in research literature, possibly because underlying assumptions have excluded this group from study. For example, it may be thought that students who were academically eligible to qualify for graduate school did not find it necessary to cheat as undergraduates. Or, graduate students may be seen as more dedicated to scholarliness and, therefore, truly interested in education for the sake of learning. The influence of age or academic maturity may account for any drop in academic dishonesty in graduate students. In a study examining 161 undergraduates and 83 graduate students in allied health programs, Falleur (1990) found a significant difference ($p < .004$) in the incidence of cheating or recent cheating behaviors and history of having cheated in high school ($p < .002$). Still, educators believe that the incidence of academic dishonesty in graduate students may be almost as great as with undergraduates (Payne & Nantz, 1994).

Sims (1993) investigated school-related and work-related dishonest behaviors in 60 students enrolled in a graduate-level business course. 91% of the subjects indicated they had participated in some form of academic dishonesty as undergraduates, and 98% had engaged in work-related dishonesty, ranging from theft or falsification to unethical practices such as preferential treatment and personal use of company time.

A survey of graduate students at a large research university (Bradshaw, 1989) identified numerous instances of academic dishonesty. The nature of the survey was to identify the prevalence of academic dishonesty and to discover if these behaviors were carried over into graduate work. The subjects ($N = 44$) were from a variety of fields: engineering, sciences, law, nursing, arts, and education. Of the group, 57% reported having participated in some form of academic dishonesty. Interestingly, nine subjects had helped a fellow student cheat or plagiarize or indicated they would do so. This clearly has ramifications for major graduate work such as research, theses, and dissertations. The likelihood for engaging in subsequent dishonest or unethical acts has been supported in research regarding business graduates in the work setting (Sims, 1993).

Professional Students. Students in professional programs can be divided into two major groups—graduate and undergraduate. As distinct groups, undergraduate students of health professions have received as little attention as have graduate students in non–health care fields. Falleur (1990) investigated perceptions of dishonest behaviors in undergraduate and graduate students in a school of health professions. Falleur only examined classroom situations and made no comparisons with clinical behaviors; therefore, his conclusions were similar to those found in studies regarding students in general education programs.

Hilbert's work (1987) with senior nursing students at four universities ($N = 210$) produced results very similar to findings reported on undergraduates in other studies. Specifically, the most commonly reported behaviors were plagiarism (51.9%), padding a bibliography (39%), giving exam answers (20.5%), and receiving exam answers (17%). Hilbert also addressed unethical clinical behaviors and received rather high reports of involvement in unprofessional acts: discussing patients in nonprofessional situations (73%), taking hospital equipment or clothes for personal use (47.6%), calling in sick when not (34%), and recording a medication that was not administered or a treatment or observation that was not done (25.7%). Hilbert (1985) reported a rise in certain behaviors over a similar study conducted at a different institution just 2 years previously. She found an increase in plagiarism, padding, and the exchange of exam answers, which also have been identified as the most common unethical behaviors. Personal unprofessional behaviors had dramatically increased, with increases in calling in sick (up 22.3%) and discussing patients (up 29.7%). Fortunately, there were decreases in the incidences of taking hospital equipment (down 11.4%) and taking medications for personal use (down 1.8%).

Daniel, Adams, and Smith (1994) sought to describe the relationship between neutralization, as described by Haines et al. (1986), maturity or commitment, and academic misconduct in nursing students. These investigators surveyed associate and bachelor's degree nursing students ($N = 190$) regarding their perceptions of their peers, rather than themselves. Subjects were asked to identify to what extent they believed peers were likely to be involved in dishonest or unethical acts, based upon such variables as age, marital status, academic ability, and academic commitment (as described by the phrase "serious students"). Two survey instruments with internal consistency were used to measure academic and clinical misconduct. Daniel et al. identified academic misconduct as cheating both on tests or assignments and outside of class, use of illegal resources, and mutilation of materials, a variable that was unique to this study but not defined by the authors. The investigators used a multivariate technique of canonical correlation analysis to examine the data. The only significant coefficient was between the variables of neutralization and maturity/commitment when accounting for variance in misconduct scores. Daniel and colleagues (1994) concluded that maturity and commitment were not perceived as associated with academic misconduct. The authors of this article also endeavored to develop a model to explain academic misconduct based upon Needs–Goal Motivation model behaviors as a precursor to a neutralizing attitude.

Sheer (1989) investigated the relationship of personality characteristics (autonomy, empathy, and socialization) as predictors of unethical classroom and clinical behaviors in nursing students ($N = 308$). Whereas these characteristics were not predictive of unethical classroom behaviors, they were predictive of unethical clinical acts. More specifically, low socialization and low autonomy were most closely linked with low moral conduct. This report is in keeping with previously cited research among undergraduate students in other fields (Anderson & Obenshain, 1994; Hetherington & Feldman, 1964; Roig & Neaman, 1994) that links the propensity toward dishonesty with alienation and feeling less self-sufficient.

Academic dishonesty in graduate professional students (dental and medical) has been investigated more thoroughly than in graduate students in other fields. Whereas medical students have reported engaging in some form of cheating, this incidence (ranging from 27% to 58% of students) seems to decrease as education advances (Rozance, 1991). In a study involving 2,459 second-year medical students from 31 different schools, Baldwin et al. (1996) concluded that 39% of the subjects had witnessed an act of cheating during their first year of medical school, yet only 4.7% reported that they had cheated. Findings in this research echoed other findings, such as a decline in frequency of academic misconduct as students advance in school. As did other investigators, Baldwin et al. concluded that the strongest predictors of academic dishonesty were previous dishonest behaviors and environmentally conducive factors. Baldwin et al. (1996) also determined that cheating was more likely among male students. This finding could be a function of gender distribution, just as in Hilbert's (1985, 1987) studies with nursing students. No other relationships between cheating and medical school students' characteristics were supported. However, Baldwin et al.'s study was limited to second-year medical students, who had not yet engaged in professional clinical situations.

Research by Anderson and Obenshain (1994) supported findings by Baldwin et al. (1996) and other researchers, especially in recounting cheating on examinations as the most common dishonest behavior. Responses by 174 medical students at a state university showed that 60% of the subjects had personal knowledge that cheating had taken place on an examination, either the giving or the receiving of information. Other outstanding findings were unauthorized group work (32%) and using a false excuse to delay an exam (11.8%).

Dishonesty in the Clinical Setting. In shifting from the didactic to the applied setting, students may feel even more challenged if they do not have a strong knowledge base. Odum (1991) pointed out that cheaters take shortcuts to passing without acquiring the knowledge and skills necessary to be competent practitioners. The self-esteem of these students is threatened and they are more apt to rely on defense mechanisms, such as rationalization, for survival. Additionally, these students may realize the importance of the information that they chose to acquire through cheating rather than studying, intensifying the threat of failure.

The psychological justification held by the cheating individual predisposes that person to engage in dishonest or unethical behaviors in the clinical setting. Previous episodes of cheating by medical students seem to be a strong predictor for subsequent dishonest acts (Baldwin et al., 1996; Falleur, 1990). Typical dishonest clinical behaviors in medical students are copying or falsifying information on a patient history and physical examination and reporting a clinical finding without obtaining the information (Anderson & Obenshain, 1994; Rozance, 1991), and these behaviors have been significantly correlated with cheating in medical school classes. Falsification on patient records by nursing students also has been reported by Hilbert (1987), along with theft and breach of confidentiality. Theft of $10 worth of items from the clinic by dental students was identified by Westerman et al. (1996) as prevalent, and 20.7% of respondents ($N = 312$) considered this not cheating or trivial cheating.

These perspectives on professional integrity have serious implications for students as they prepare for transition into independent professional practice. Students who adopt a cavalier or nonchalant attitude about honesty in academic situations display behavioral patterns that will emerge in other settings as well. Furthermore, students cheat or commit other fraudulent acts in order to continue in their educational programs are not thoroughly grounded in the knowledge base needed for practice. Ozar (1991) indicated that cheating on tests is a form of misrepresentation: Dishonest students are attempting to portray that they know as much as honest students. Gaberson (1997) pointed out that students who misrepresent themselves, such as using assistance calculating a medication dosage, leave the faculty and/or preceptor with the impression that they are capable of this skill as well as other forms of problem solving. In relating misrepresentation to professional behaviors, Ozar (1991) and Odum (1991) maintained that dishonest students will likely misrepresent their competency as practitioners.

Attitudes Toward Academic Dishonesty: Students and Faculty

Students. The number of incidences of academic dishonesty and the contributing psychological factors directly reflect the attitudes held by students on all levels—undergraduate, graduate, and professional. Dishonest students who graduate and continue to misrepresent themselves in practice can reflect poorly upon their educational program. Students and graduates do not want to work with someone who is underprepared and dishonest about work (Gaberson, 1997).

Personal achievement and successful completion of educational programs have a higher value to some students than do commitment to institutional standards and expectations (Nuss, 1984). Sims (1993) concluded that choosing to participate in academic dishonesty reflects a student's attitude, and this attitude toward dishonesty will be translated to other aspects of life. This can be exemplified by the relationship between dishonest acts and low organizational affiliation, especially with large organizations. Students on campuses at larger universities have less compunction about cheating because they feel less responsible to the institution and its codes of behavior (Fishbein, 1994). Competition, personal gratification, and goals may explain why business majors are more likely to approve of and participate in cheating than are liberal arts majors (Baird, 1980). Odum (1991) went further to say that students develop low morale about their work and low values about their profession when they realize that selected goals can be realized dishonestly, rather than through hard work. Cheating and plagiarism become easy to justify, especially because small percentages of research subjects (1.3% of sample) report ever having been caught (Haines et al., 1986). Much of this comes from the trust that dishonest students place in peers to not report them (McCabe & Trevino, 1993), an additional lapse in ethics.

Situational ethics, as described by Anderson and Obenshain (1994), can excuse participation in academic dishonesty in certain situations. In fact, students have indicated that their acts of dishonesty are in retaliation to faculty who "cheat" them by ineffective teaching, using underprepared graduate assistants, missing classes, and focusing on research rather than on teaching and students (Fishbein, 1994). Conversely, greater faculty involvement with students and commitment to maintaining academic integrity produce a low incidence of cheating or plagiarism (Anderson & Obenshain, 1994).

It is encouraging to note that as students improve their academic standing, they are more inclined to disapprove of cheating and to agree with faculty about enforcing disciplinary measures (Sims, 1995). Hawley (1984) reported a victimization response from honest students, in that they feel cheated by having to compete with dishonest students for better work, which may explain a lower tolerance of academic dishonesty especially among more advanced students. In professional students, there seems to be agreement that cheating is rarely justified (Warman, Harvan, & Weidman, 1994; Westerman et. al., 1996). Research by Westerman and colleagues revealed a more serious approach toward dishonesty as students progressed from undergraduate to professional studies. In these students, peer pressure, the preprofessional link with future peer review, seemed to be effective in discouraging unethical acts. Interestingly, the one instance in which dishonesty was justifiable among these students was to protect themselves or others from lawsuit, a new moral dimension that emerges from professional education (Warman et al., 1994; Westerman et al., 1996).

Regarding formal disciplinary measures, published research indicates that students' attitudes regarding a printed or announced honor code and penalties for academic dishonesty are mixed. Whereas there is agreement that students respond positively to faculty announcing or discussing the honor code, cheating, plagiarism, and penalties (Anderson & Obenshain, 1994; McCabe & Trevino, 1993; Sheer, 1989), some authors believe that a published announcement on these matters has little influence on students' attitudes and actions (Fossbinder, 1991). For students who continue to cheat in the face of announced penalties, there is a strong association with acts of cheating since high school (Davis & Ludvigson, 1995). Thus, announcement of penalties seems to not deter planned cheating in students who have long been involved in such behaviors.

In a large study ($N = 6,096$, 31 sites), McCabe and Trevino (1993) determined that self-reported cheating was higher among students at institutions that did not have an honor code. In the entire sample, peer behavior had the greatest influence, both positively and negatively, on academic honesty. The authors also concluded that cheating and similar behaviors may be learned from peers, and many actions, especially those related to the situation, may occur as the result of peer input.

Faculty. Even though faculty are aware of the existence of cheating, lying, and plagiarism, they are generally reluctant to accept the fact that it occurs in their own classes. Being in a professional milieu based upon a strong ethical code, faculty may be surprised that the milieu attracts students who do not have a strong code of personal ethics (Anderson & Obenshain, 1994). The discrepancy in views is exemplified by the numerous studies that have indicated a lack of agreement between students and faculty on what constitutes academic dishonesty.

Bailey (1990) found a discrepancy between faculty beliefs regarding acts of cheating or plagiarism and descriptions of such instances. Bailey surveyed 262 nursing faculty and education administrators who were chairs or deans of nursing programs. Her design was structured specifically to receive responses from both faculty and administrators in order to examine consensus between these groups. The administrators were asked to complete a questionnaire plus distribute a questionnaire to a faculty member who had more than three years of teaching experience and to a faculty member who had less than three years of experience. The survey addressed four areas of concern: perception about what constituted cheating, whether cheating was a problem in the subject's program, perception of colleague support when confronting a student who cheated, and a description of a critical incident in which cheating or plagiarism occurred and how the problem was solved. 61% of the faculty and 46% of the administrators did not perceive cheating as a problem. Years of teaching experience did not influence the results; 69% percent of the faculty with less than three years in teaching did not believe cheating was a problem, in agreement with 61% of faculty with more than three years of experience. 92% of the subjects indicated that their programs had administrative policies regarding cheating and plagiarism; however, 25% of these subjects also indicated that they believed their policies to be ineffective. This response was similar to faculty responses in Carmack's (1984) study.

When faculty had to impose disciplinary action because of cheating or plagiarism, 97% of Bailey's (1990) sample perceived administrators to be supportive of the faculty member involved in the case. Faculty did perceive, however, that administrators were more supportive than fellow faculty in such instances. 60% of the subjects could describe a critical incident in which cheating or plagiarism had occurred and how they dealt with the incident. In most cases, the administrative policies were enforced, but some faculty described situations in which the dishonest student was allowed to continue in the nursing program. The reporting of critical incidents seems incongruous with the subjects' perception that cheating is not a problem. Bailey did not define the word "problem" in her report of this study, so it is unclear how the subjects interpreted this word. It is possible that even though many of the subjects had been involved in situations of cheating or plagiarism by students and knew that dishonest acts occur, the faculty believed that those situations could be resolved effectively. On the other hand, faculty and administrators may be underestimating the number of acts of academic dishonesty.

In light of the faculty role to uphold professional and educational standards, there are some interesting attitudes among faculty regarding school honor codes and discipline for dishonest acts. Even in institutions with clearly defined policies, many faculty choose not to follow the guidelines but deal with academic dishonesty on a personal level (i.e., "one-to-one") (McCabe & Trevino, 1993). Odum (1991) indicated that faculty who choose to not implement disciplinary measures (proctoring, punishment, etc.) do so because such measures are paternalistic, authoritarian, and, therefore, displeasing and in opposition to the framework of professional relationships. Carmack (1984) found that many nursing faculty do not want to be the "bad guy." Also, faculty reluctance can come from lack of sufficient information to support disciplinary measures (Falleur, 1990). Nuss (1984) pointed out that merely assigning a failing grade serves as little punishment to a student who was in jeopardy of failing anyway. Furthermore, this penalty does not enable students to actually confront underlying causes of unacceptable academic behavior. In research interviews with 21 nursing faculty, Carmack (1984) discovered that many subjects would be lenient with acts of plagiarism, giving students a second chance or selecting disciplinary measures based upon the seriousness of the assignment and the extent of plagiarism. In other words faculty seem to perceive some gray areas of moral conduct.

For faculty who are frustrated by continued academic dishonesty, often the difficulty in dealing with cheating stems from a lack of administrative support or a cumbersome due-process mechanism. In describing perspectives on plagiarism, probably one of the most difficult forms of dishonesty to prove (in terms of intent), Skom (1986) noted, "While the university community speaks strongly against plagiarism, it does not always follow through on the principles it advocates" (p. 88). Carmack's (1984) research supported this dilemma, citing that many of her subjects did not want to get entangled in a legal process that seemed to favor the students. Hopelessness, helplessness, and resignation to the problem are attitudes that faculty held when faced with the long-standing, complex problems of fraud and deceit in education.

Legal Implications

Helms and Weiler (1991) examined litigation patterns in nursing education. The authors surveyed state and federal case law from 1961 through 1989 and found that only 24 cases were linked to nursing education. Of that number, nine cases were initiated by students who were disputing dismissal from the program. Only one case was identified by the authors as being related to dismissal because of student cheating. Although the outcome of that case was not reported, students did prevail in the majority of cases in which they brought suit. The most frequent claim was a violation of due process. Helm and Weiler cautioned that although the number of cases reported in case law is low, the number of cases that are filed and dismissed or settled is much higher. In addition, a limitation of the study was that state court system cases only report appeals cases, so that the actual number of cases adjudicated in the state system is not known.

Denial of due process in academic dishonesty cases as a reason for filing lawsuits is also demonstrated in the selected case law described by Kaplin and Lee (1995) and by Olivas (1989). Student claims were rejected when the university was found to have provided students an opportunity to respond to charges against them and to be heard by an impartial grievance panel (*Gorman v. University of Rhode Island*, as cited in Kaplin & Lee, 1995; *Jaska v. Regents of the University of Michigan*, as cited in Kaplin & Lee, 1995). Olivas (1989) noted that there have been differences in verdicts on the need for legal counsel in student hearings. Dismissal was reversed in a precedent-setting case due to failure of the university to allow the student to have legal counsel at a disciplinary hearing (*University of Houston v. Sabeti*, as cited in Olivas, 1989). However, succeeding cases have held to a less rigid system, when the institution had written procedures in place and the courts determined that expulsion hearing did not require confrontation and cross-examination of witness (*Greenhill v. Bailey*, as cited in Olivas, 1989; *Goss v. Lopez*, as cited in Olivas, 1989).

Although fear of being sued may cause concern in faculty who wish to pursue cases of academic dishonesty, establishment and implementation of due-process procedures have been demonstrated to be the best defense against student claims of unfair treatment (Helms & Weiler, 1991; Kaplin & Lee, 1995; Olivas, 1989). None of the cases reviewed were based on allegations of slander, although these studies did not report all cases filed. The major findings were that faculty need to document that the student was offered an opportunity to tell his or her side of the story and that the grievance process was carried out appropriately.

STRATEGIES FOR PREVENTING AND DEALING WITH ACADEMIC DISHONESTY

Most of the literature on prevention and procedures for dealing with academic dishonesty is case-based and provides procedural recommendations (Bradshaw & Lowenstein, 1990; Carmack, 1984; Saunders, 1993; Wilholt, 1994). There is little research on the effectiveness of the suggested strategies for addressing this problem. Strategies have been developed based on studies of causative factors (Barnett & Dalton, 1981; Genereux & McLeod, 1995). Tables 4–1 through 4–4 are a compendium of strategies suggested in the literature (Booth & Hoyer, 1992; Bradshaw & Lowenstein, 1990; Davis, Johnston, DiMicco, Findlay, & Taylor, 1996; Saunders, 1993; Wilhoit, 1994).

TABLE 4–1.
Preventing Academic Dishonesty

1. Inform students of the importance of the issues of cheating, plagiarism, and unethical professional behavior early in the program and reinforce in individual course syllabi. This may be done through classroom discussion and distribution of polices or defining statements. Include the following:
   - Review the conventions of citing references, quoting sources, and validating ideas.
   - Define and discuss plagiarism and unauthorized collaboration.
   - Distribute and discuss school polices regarding plagiarism, including penalties.
   - Explain specific regulations, which could include a requirement to include a previous draft of a paper with the final paper or submission of photocopies of documented material or articles.

2. To reduce the opportunity for cheating, exam proctors must be alert and visible, and sufficient space must be allotted between exam takers. Students must be made aware that faculty view cheating as a serious offense. Use of past examination material should be minimized and test security maintained. Rules for take-home exams should be explicitly defined.

3. Be aware of student workloads and consider alternatives to planned assignments in order to reduce excessive workloads.

4. Establish a nonpunitive climate for honest mistakes that includes using mistakes as learning opportunities.

5. Be prepared to deal with a case of suspected fraud, by understanding and periodically reviewing institutional policies regarding academic dishonesty.

TABLE 4–2.
Identifying Academic Dishonesty

1. Be alert to inappropriate or uncharacteristic behaviors.

2. Gather and analyze evidence to distinguish between dishonest intent and ignorance of appropriate behavior and to analyze for patterns.

3. Thoroughly document suspect behaviors, including date, time, and names of witnesses to the behavior. Be sure any statements by students or witnesses are submitted voluntarily; involved faculty may need to assign a neutral party to collect such statements. Document conversations with the student clarifying behaviors.

4. Develop a clear understanding of the circumstances under which cheating should be formally reported.

5. Develop appropriate administrative support to carry the incident further.

TABLE 4–3.
Procedures Once Academic Dishonesty Has Been Identified

1. Maintain consistency among faculty when imposing sanctions related to academic dishonesty.

2. Notify the student of the charge and the source of the charge.

3. Once formal action has been instituted, give the student a copy of the procedure that will be followed.

4. Depending on institutional procedures, the student may be permitted to confront or cross-examine witnesses and may have the right to a hearing and legal or advocacy representation.

5. Make the student aware of the appeal process.

TABLE 4–4.
Postincident Strategies

1. Evaluate the process and outcome to provide opportunity for revision of outdated or ineffective policies.

2. Schedule faculty education sessions to help faculty reach consensus about approaches to academic dishonesty.

Booth and Hoyer (1992) promoted an ethical approach to handling academic dishonesty that relies on faculty autonomy and students' rights to presumed innocence and due process. The faculty is held to the principles of "beneficence" and "nonmaleficence." The situation must be used to stimulate the student's moral development without compromising the rights of any other involved person or patient. The authors noted that universities or colleges and schools of nursing should have published policies to deal with academic dishonesty and to define due process. In addition, health care facilities should have written standards of practice that can impact clinical experiences, of which faculty and students need to be aware.

For cases of failed integrity, Booth and Hoyer (1992) developed a decision tree that provides an overview of actions that faculty can take. Once a complaint is registered, fact-finding is instituted, which includes interviews with involved parties and written documentation. An informal hearing may be held and a decision made regarding the seriousness of the complaint. At this point, a decision is made whether the complaint is considered minor, moderate, or severe, and different strategies may be implemented. Minor incidents may bring about a reprimand and possible rehabilitative action. Moderate incidents may include a lowered or failing mark and rehabilitative actions that may include additional fact-finding and sanctions, with opportunity for student appeal. Severe infringements may lead to suspension or dismissal and may require additional fact-finding and a formal hearing; an appeal may occur. Whether the incident is minor, moderate, or major, the incident is documented in the student's record.

Consistency among faculty and consistency in sanctions are important in handling academic dishonesty. Bailey's (1990) research with nursing faculty indicates the value of perceived support from colleagues and consistent policy application from administrators when addressing academic dishonesty. Consistency is an important aspect of the decision to bring official or formal action or to keep the incident informal, solely between instructor and student. Awareness of different treatment may impact the perception of fairness and impartiality and can trigger a distrustful climate; inconsistency may also be grounds for appeal.

DISCUSSION OF RESEARCH LITERATURE

Many investigators (Barnett & Dalton, 1981; Falleur, 1990; Hawley, 1984; Nuss, 1984; Peterson, 1986; Roth & McCabe, 1995; Skom, 1986; Uhlig & Howes, 1967) reported two underlying, related problems that could contribute to the incidence or causes of academic dishonesty. First, faculty and students did not agree on what constituted academic fraud and the related penalty. Second, student subjects genuinely did not understand acts that constituted academic dishonesty, especially plagiarism and authorized collaboration. Many college catalogs did not print academic dishonesty policies (Weaver, Davis, Look, Bizzanga, & Neal, 1991). At these institutions, it is possible that guidelines are not set down for students, or that guidelines and accompanying penalties are individualized by faculty and course. Lack of clarity about what constitutes academic dishonesty may arise, and students might see ethical standards as the idiosyncrasy of one professor. Mawdsley (1985) believes that faculty are obligated to define and give examples of plagiarism, in order to provide a fair warning of expectations.

The literature reviewed demonstrates that there are many intentional thoughts and much conscious awareness associated with academic dishonesty, especially cheating and lying. Excuse making and personal justification, along with situational ethics, seem to be the driving forces behind deceitful behaviors. The neutralization theory (Haines et al., 1986) explains why students excuse and/or permit cheating in others. In contrast to observations linking extracurricular activities and increased incidence of cheating (Haines et al., 1986), Baird (1980) noted that students who participate more in extracurricular activities are more likely to disapprove of cheating. Whereas types of extracurricular activities varied from study to study, they are best contrasted as socially oriented versus service oriented. Students involved in socially oriented activities, such as sports or sororities, also tended to be younger and less serious about their education. Students in service-oriented endeavors, such as student government, were more enmeshed in the academic culture and placed higher value on its standards. These students, as a group, disapproved of cheating and supported disciplinary measures. This finding was supported by Davis and Ludvigson (1995), who believe that more involvement in the educational process yields a stronger commitment to academic integrity and the purposes of higher education. Students who operate on a higher or more sophisticated level of moral reasoning are less likely to engage in academic dishonesty because of the inability to develop personal justification for such acts (Barnett & Dalton, 1981).

Regarding design and methodology of studies on academic dishonesty, at least two potential weaknesses can be identified. First, the sensitive nature of the topic and the faculty–student relationship imposes certain limitations on subject selection and research questions. Investigators can draw conclusions from results but have no opportunity to validate the findings with subjects. As in other types of studies, findings are limited by the questions asked. Second, due to the moral character of potential subjects, there is great opportunity for deceit, even on the questionnaires. In other words, there is a possibility that cheaters and liars falsified their answers on research instruments. Students' suspicions may have altered results; conversely, it is possible that students used the studies as an opportunity to confess transgressions. Also, these studies provided self-reported data that cannot be verified. No studies exist that describe observed clinical behaviors, such as falsifying patient records or theft.

Of the studies in this review, there are other limitations regarding subject selection. Investigators have reported an increase in moral development and a subsequent decrease in academic dishonesty with academically mature students, such as those in upper division or graduate programs (Baird, 1980; Falleur, 1990; Haines et al., 1986). However, Hilbert (1985, 1987) surveyed only senior nursing students, who had more clinical experience and presumably more moral development than their junior peers, yet she reported many dishonest classroom and clinical acts. Nursing educators should be cautious in generalizing Hilbert's findings to other nursing programs, since sophomore and junior students were not included for comparison. Also, if Hilbert's subjects, as more mature learners, are indicative of more advanced moral development as described in other studies, the reader is uncertain about the level of integrity in less mature learners.

Daniel et al. (1994) developed conclusions based upon perceived behaviors of peers rather than reported observations (as in studies by Anderson & Obenshain, 1994, and Baldwin et al., 1996). The authors' stated purpose was to develop background information that could be used as a framework for interventions for dealing with academic misconduct. Given the complex nature of the research reported in their article, Daniel and colleagues might have acquired more significant data if they had surveyed subjects' views of themselves rather than of others.

Many of the studies cited in this chapter used convenience samples of students available on investigators' campuses (Anderson & Obenshain, 1994; Bradshaw, 1989; Falluer, 1990; Hilbert, 1985, 1987; Warman et al., 1994; Westerman et al., 1996). Some investigators were even more selective by using students from their own courses as subjects (Hetherington & Feldman, 1964; Payne & Nantz, 1994; Sims, 1993; Uhlig & Howes, 1967). Some of these are earlier studies that were foundational to describing the problems of academic dishonesty. More recent students have broadened their scope, in terms of sample size, to better generalize findings.

Seventeen of the studies reviewed were descriptive studies using survey questionnaires. Whereas this may limit the scope of the problem of academic dishonesty, it does facilitate comparison of findings from study to study. Some of the articles reviewed included information about established validity of survey instruments. In one of the published studies, authors reported pretesting the survey instrument (Anderson & Obenshain, 1994). Falleur (1990) established content validity based upon agreement among educators about definitions of terms used in the questionnaire; this is an interesting approach to content validity, since Falleur's findings revealed that faculty and students differed in their definitions of plagiarism. A possible discrepancy in beliefs may explain Falleur's findings yet weakens the content validity. Hilbert (1985) defined dishonest behavior in the classroom from a review of literature on the subject. Similarly to Falleur, Hilbert (1985) asked faculty to define unethical clinical behaviors, and she indicated that content validity on both terms was assumed. Hilbert used the same instrument in a subsequent study (1987), and thus agreement between the findings of her two studies can be reached. Both Hilbert and Falleur reported internal consistency. Falleur (1990) used alpha coefficient for internal consistency ($\alpha = .77$), as did Hilbert (1985) ($\alpha = .668$), but Hilbert pointed out that coefficient alpha might not be appropriate for her criterion-referenced scale. Daniel et al. (1994) reported internal consistency on scales or subscales used but did not provide coefficients.

Other investigators used descriptive statistics, such as percentages, *t* test, Pearson correlation coefficients, and analysis of variance (ANOVA), to characterize their findings (Baldwin et al., 1996; Bradshaw, 1989; Sheer, 1989; Warman et al., 1994; Westerman et al., 1996). Daniel and colleagues (1994) used canonical correlation analysis to examine multiple predictors in combination with multiple criteria. Anderson and Obenshain (1994) employed chi-square to describe findings between faculty and students regarding unethical behaviors. Westerman et al. (1996) used chi-square to examine beliefs among dental students, in the first two years and the last two years of their programs, on response to cheating; the authors examined whether students reported cheating and how they rated the severity of different types of cheating. Baldwin and colleagues (1996) used a contingency table with their large sample ($N = 3,975$) to score perceived ethical standard in self and rating of severity of cheating.

It is unfortunate that so few studies exist regarding nursing students. A review of literature in professional education identified more studies on medical or dental students, and many studies were published since 1990. These studies were exclusively survey through questionnaire, thus presenting the limitations of self-reporting. The research publications that were directed at undergraduate nursing students were limited to convenience samples but had adequate samples. Research with nursing faculty (two studies) used questionnaire, interview, and critical incident methods. No studies in medicine or dentistry used qualitative methods. Table 4–5 provides an overview of the research studies ($N = 10$) on professional students, both graduate and undergraduate.

TABLE 4–5.
Research on Academic Dishonesty in Professional Students

Author	Subjects	Study Design	Findings
Anderson & Obenshain (1994)	174 medical students and 206 medical school faculty.	Descriptive survey.	Agreement between faculty and students about effectiveness of honor code and seriousness of cheating on exams; both faculty and students engaged in situational ethics regarding practice-related decisions.
Bailey (1990)	242 nursing faculty.	Descriptive questionnaire and critical incident description.	Faculty did not perceive cheating as a problem. Colleagues were supportive in cheating situations.

TABLE 4–5.
Research on Academic Dishonesty in Professional Students (Continued)

Author	Subjects	Study Design	Findings
Baldwin et al. (1996)	2,459 medical students.	Descriptive survey.	Episodes of cheating in medical school witnessed by 39% of respondents; honor codes held only small effect over cheating; best predictor of cheating was previous experiences in cheating.
Daniel et al. (1994)	Associate and bachelor's degree nursing students.	Descriptive opinion survey.	Students perceived less likelihood of academic misconduct in peers who were married, were more serious about academics, and were more able to do academic work.
Falleur (1990)	83 graduate students, 166 undergraduate students, and 31 faculty in a school of health professionals.	Descriptive survey.	Faculty and students differed in definitions of plagiarism; 30% of student subjects had cheated in college; cheating was more frequent in male students; fewer incidences of cheating were reported by graduate students.
Hilbert (1985)	101 senior nursing students.	Descriptive survey.	Subjects reported lower incidences of unethical classroom behaviors and a higher percentage of agreement on what was unethical when compared to larger sample of general education students; significant relationship $(p < .001)$ between unethical classroom and clinical behaviors was found.

TABLE 4–5.
Research on Academic Dishonesty in Professional Students (Continued)

Author	Subjects	Study Design	Findings
Hilbert (1987)	210 senior nursing students.	Descriptive survey.	Using same instrument as in 1985 study, discovered a rise in unethical behaviors in both class and clinical work as well as a significant relationship ($P = .00000$) between the two variables.
Sheer (1989)	308 nursing students.	Descriptive survey; scales measuring socialization, autonomy, and empathy.	Personality profiles could not predict unethical classroom behaviors but were predictive of unethical clinical behaviors. Academic policies were deterrents to unethical behaviors.
Warman et al. (1994)	243 dental students.	Descriptive survey.	Giving or receiving help was not perceived as serious cheating; some percentages of students could justify cheating, especially in lawsuit situations.
Westerman et al. (1996)	292 dental students.	Descriptive survey (used a revised version of Warman's instrument).	Subjects identified many situations, including theft of clinic items, as not serious; some justification among subjects for cheating, either in lawsuits or to get even with a teacher; 55% of subjects would report cheating.

To apply research findings on academic dishonesty in higher education to nursing students, basic assumptions are needed. It must be assumed that nursing students, especially those in associate and baccalaureate degree programs, are homogenous with the general population of undergraduate college students. In fact, most nursing students take introductory or lower division coursework with the general student population. Hilbert's two studies (1985, 1987) with nursing students indicated that these students did not differ from the general population of college students. It also must be assumed that nursing students have the same academic goals, challenges, and problems as do other students: desire for good grades, fear of failure, work and other priorities, need for socialization, and financial pressures. Consequently, conclusions about the causes and incidences of academic dishonesty should not exclude nursing students. Opportunistic cheating, unauthorized collaboration, padding of bibliographies, or lying about results on clinical papers may occur in nursing programs. Gender may be an issue, since nursing programs are female-dominated; studies indicate that there is a greater tendency for male students to cheat, and that female students are more responsive to announced penalties for cheating (Davis & Ludvigson, 1995; Falleur, 1990; Genereux & McLeod, 1995).

There is the potential that nursing students, especially younger ones, who continue to affiliate with social groups rather than nursing organizations are less likely to identify with the nursing program, and professional standards. The need to work collaboratively and be part of the group, plus the pressure of a rigorous program could initiate the use of defense mechanisms and other psychological attitudes associated with cheating. The confounding of poor professional socialization, a career goal of obtaining a degree in nursing, and subsequent need to pass the National Council Licensure Examination (NCLEX) could cause the student to be very fearful of failure. Being enrolled in more relevant coursework, along with academic maturity, causes students to see less reason to cheat (Payne & Nantz, 1994). Daniel et al. (1994) explained the concept of neutralization among nursing students by pointing out that nurses often are viewed as role models of integrity. For a nursing student involved in academic dishonesty, neutralization may be a mechanism by which one can maintain an outwardly honest image while simultaneously compromising one's own integrity.

McCabe and Bowers (1994) predicted that plagiarism and the padding of bibliographies will decrease, due to the availability of rapidly accessible on-line reference sources and other technological advances. Many databases are full text, which easily provide students with supportive documentation for assigned papers. On the other hand, computer-literate students may discover numerous creative ways to falsify written assignments. For examples, access to on-line databases enables users to select any number of documents for bibliographic reference without actually reading the sources. Full text articles, especially those which are research based, can be plagiarized from the database as easily as they can from the published journal or book. It is even likely that students can plagiarize from obscure sources or those not readily available to faculty for scrutiny. Faculty will need to include means to validate sources as part of the assignment; requiring printed copies of sources would be an easy way to conduct this validation. As faculty develop computerized testing for course exams, safeguards against access to the answers or a fellow student's test need to be included in the system.

IMPLICATIONS FOR NURSING EDUCATION

Professional misconduct has serious implications for the novice nurse. When students or beginning practitioners see fellow students and colleagues falsify documentation about patients, take shortcuts, steal, or lie, a delicate moral framework is damaged. Confusion sets in and the novice falls into the dilemma of situational ethics, excuse making, and similar tactics. Guidance by established professionals who are able to direct moral development and decision making clearly is needed (Hoyer, Booth, Spelman, & Richardson, 1991). Sims (1993) asserted that adults (i.e., faculty), should insist on students' responsibility for their own behaviors and the accompanying moral obligations. Professional misconduct, like plagiarism, may arise in beginning students from a lack of procedural knowledge rather than the intent to deceive. Still, correct guidelines for action must be taught and reinforced.

An honor code policy deters dishonest behavior in the classroom. Sheer's (1989) findings regarding incidences of unethical or dishonest behaviors in clinical settings among students who have an honor code policy for the classroom indicate conflicting attitudes toward such codes. One might conclude that the subjects in this study upheld academic standards only when guidelines for behavior and the related penalties were made clear. The study certainly suggests that guidelines regarding ethical behaviors in clinical settings are not clear or that violations go unpunished.

The subjects in Hilbert's 1987 study indicated that the most common excuse for unethical clinical behaviors was that the behaviors "did not seem unethical." The responsibility to communicate what constitutes appropriate professional behaviors clearly lies with faculty. Faculty must preserve their own integrity as well. To allow students who are chronic cheaters and liars to enter into practice reflects poorly on the professional program and its faculty. Acts of plagiarism that go undetected may later appear in a publication by the student. Faculty, as advisors or collaborators, might then be liable for violations of copyright law (Mawdsley, 1985).

RECOMMENDATIONS FOR FURTHER STUDY

This chapter analyzed existing studies regarding the many aspects of academic dishonesty. It is curious that there are so few studies regarding this problem in nursing education. Although the literature reviewed indicates a strong likelihood that nursing students do, at some point, encounter academic dishonesty while in college, there are no recent studies examining the certainty or magnitude of this problem. There also have been no studies since 1990 that describe faculty perceptions regarding academic dishonesty and administrative support when problems arise. Furthermore, available studies regarding faculty perceptions of incidences of cheating or plagiarism show that faculty may actually underestimate the extent of the problem. Research addressing these issues, with a current look at dishonest and unethical behaviors as well as an emphasis on solutions to the problems, is warranted. Of special interest would be research directed toward the link between perceived dishonest behaviors and perceived unethical practices among students and novice nurses.

Replication of studies should be conducted with nursing students. For example, an investigation of the relationship between printed policies (see Weaver et al., 1991) or honor codes (see McCabe & Trevino, 1993) and incidences of cheating might reveal to what extent such policies deter cheating. An observational study such as the one conducted by Hetherington and Feldman (1964) could reveal actual practices by nursing students when placed in situations conducive to cheating. Clinical faculty might observe ethically challenging situations in patient care settings and thereby update knowledge on dishonesty in the work setting as reported by Anderson and Obenshain (1994), Hilbert (1987), and Westerman et al. (1996).

None of the available studies used a qualitative method with nursing students. Such studies could yield rich data that might help faculty prevent or confront the problems in academic dishonesty. A qualitative researcher could develop an interview aimed at gleaning nursing students' perspectives on such topics as efficacy of honor codes, actual knowledge of plagiarism, or beliefs about student and faculty responsibilities regarding academic and clinical ethics.

CONCLUSION

Faculty in professional programs have a responsibility to ensure that new practitioners are educationally prepared and clinically competent (Ozar, 1991). Nursing faculty, as guardians of professional education and standards, are charged with ascertaining that all students learn what is essential and necessary for practice (Carmack, 1984). Of equal importance is the role modeling of good judgment and ego strength and the willingness to take decisive action in the face of wrongdoing.

The challenge for nursing faculty is twofold: As teachers, faculty must develop effective learning environments that eliminate the perceived need to cheat. Institutions of higher education need to develop learning environments in which all forms of academic dishonesty are clearly unacceptable behaviors. As professional practitioners, faculty are charged with verifying the competency and ethical standards of the newest members of the profession. Through these endeavors, the ethical nature of the profession can be sustained.

REFERENCES

Anderson, R. E., & Obenshain, S. S. (1994). Cheating by students: Findings, reflections, and remedies. *Academic Medicine, 69*, 323–332.

Bailey, P. A. (1990). Cheating among nursing students. *Nurse Educator, 15*(3), 32–35.

Baird, J. S. (1980). Current trends in college cheating. *Psychology in the Schools, 17*, 515–522.

Baldwin, D. C., Daugherty, S. R., Rowley, B. D., & Schwarz, D. (1996). Cheating in medical school: A survey of second-year students at 31 schools. *Academic Medicine, 71*, 267–273.

Barnett, D. C., & Dalton, J. C. (1981). Why college students cheat. *Journal of College Student Personnel, 22,* 545–550.

Baumeister, R. F., & Scher, S. J. (1988). Self-defeating behavior patterns among normal individuals: Review and analysis of common self-destructive tendencies. *Psychological Bulletin, 104,* 3–22.

Booth, D. E., & Hoyer, P. J. (1992). Cheating: Faculty responsibilities when integrity fails. *Nursing Outlook, 40,* 86–93.

Bradshaw, M. J. (1989) *Academic dishonesty in graduate students.* Unpublished manuscript.

Bradshaw, M. J., & Lowenstein, A. J. (1990). Perspectives on academic dishonesty. *Nurse Educator, 15*(5), 10–15.

Carmack, B. J. (1984). Exploring nursing educators' experience with student plagiarism. *Nurse Educator, 9,* 29–33.

Daniel, L. G., Adams, B. N., & Smith, N. M. (1994). Academic misconduct among nursing students: A multivariate investigation. *Journal of Professional Nursing, 10,* 278–288.

Davis, M., Johnston, S. R., DiMicco, W., Findlay, M. P., & Taylor, J. A. (1996). The case for student honor code and beyond. *Journal of Professional Nursing, 12,* 24–30.

Davis, S. F., & Ludvigson, H. W. (1995). Additional data on academic dishonesty and a proposal for remediation. *Teaching of Psychology, 22,* 119–121.

Falleur, D. (1990). An investigation of academic dishonesty in allied health. Incidence and definitions. *Journal of Allied Health, 19,* 313–323.

Fishbein, L. (1994). We can curb college cheating. *Chronicle of Higher Education, 40,* A52.

Ford, C. V., King, B. H., & Hollender, M. H. (1988). Lies and liars: Psychiatric aspects of prevarication. *American Journal of Psychiatry, 145,* 554–562.

Fossbinder, D. (1991). Cheating and plagiarism. *Nurse Educator, 16,* 5.

Gaberson, K. B. (1997). Academic dishonesty among nursing students. *Nursing Forum, 32*(3), 14–20.

Genereux, R. L., & McLeod, B. A. (1995) Circumstances surrounding cheating: A questionnaire study of college of students. *Research in Higher Education, 36,* 687–704.

Haines, V. J., Diekhoff, G. M., LaBeff, E. E., & Clark, R. E. (1986). College cheating: Immaturity, lack of commitment, and the neutralizing attitude. *Research in Higher Education, 25,* 342–354.

Hawley, C. S. (1984). The thieves of academe: Plagiarism in the university system. *Improving College and University Teaching, 32,* 35–39.

Helms, L. B., & Weiler, K. (1991). Suing programs of nursing education. *Nursing Outlook, 30,* 158–161.

Hetherington, E. M., & Feldman, S. E. (1964). College cheating as a function of subject and situational variables. *Journal of Educational Psychology, 55,* 212–218.

Hilbert, G. A. (1985). Involvement of nursing students in unethical classroom and clinical behaviors. *Journal of Professional Nursing, 1,* 230–234.

Hilbert, G. A. (1987). Academic fraud: Prevalence, practices, and reasons. *Journal of Professional Nursing, 3,* 39–45.

Hoyer, P. J., Booth, D., Spelman, M. R., & Richardson, C. E. (1991). Clinical cheating and moral development. *Nursing Outlook, 39,* 170–173.

Kaplin, W. A., & Lee, B. A. (1995). *The law of higher education: A comprehensive guide to legal implications of academic decision making* (3rd ed.). San Francisco: Jossey Bass.

Mawdsley, R. D. (1985). *Legal aspects of plagiarism.* Topeka, KS: National Organization on Legal Problems in Education. (ERIC Document No. 268 624.)

McCabe, D. L., & Bowers, W. J. (1994). Academic dishonesty among males in college: A thirty year perspective. *Journal of College Student Development, 35,* 5–10.

McCabe, D. L., & Trevino, L. K. (1993). Academic dishonesty: Honor codes and other contextual influences. *Journal of Higher Education, 64,* 523–538.

McCabe, D. L., & Trevino, L. K. (1996). What we know about cheating in college: Longitudinal trends and recent developments. *Change, 28,* 29–33.

Nuss, E. M. (1984). Academic integrity: Comparing faculty and student attitudes. *Improving College and University Teaching, 32,* 140–144.

Odum, J. G. (1991). The practical ramifications of cheating. *Journal of Dental Education, 55,* 272–275.

Olivas, M. A. (1989). *The law and higher education: Cases and material on colleges in court.* Durham, NC: Carolina Academic Press.

Ozar, D. T. (1991) The ethical ramifications of cheating. *Journal of Dental Education, 55,* 276–281.

Payne, S. L., & Nantz, K. S. (1994). Social accounts and metaphors about cheating. *College Teaching, 42,* 90–96.

Peterson, O. (1986). "But we did it together, " or academic integrity and misrepresentation among college students. (ERIC Report No. HE 019 799; ERIC Document No. 275 281)

Roig, M., & Neaman, M. A. (1994). Alienation, learning or grade orientation, and achievement as correlates of attitudes toward cheating. *Perceptual and Motor Skills, 78,* 1096–1098.

Roth, N. L., & McCabe, D. L. (1995). Communication strategies for addressing academic dishonesty. *Journal of College Student Development, 36,* 531–541.

Rozance, C. P. (1991). Cheating in medical schools: Implications for students and patients. *Journal of the American Medical Association, 266,* 2453, 2456.

Saunders, E. J. (1993). Confronting academic dishonesty. *Journal of Social Work Education, 29,* 224–251.

Sheer, B. L. (1989). The relationships among socialization, empathy, autonomy, and unethical student behaviors in baccalaureate nursing students. *Dissertation Abstracts International, 51,* 147B.

Sims, R. (1993). The relationship between academic dishonesty and unethical business practices. *Journal of Education for Business, 68,* 207–211

Sims, R. (1995). The severity of academic dishonesty: A comparison of faculty and student views. *Psychology in the Schools, 32,* 233–238.

Skom, E. (1986). *Plagiarism: Quite a rather bad little crime* (Report No. HE 019 845). Washington, DC: American Association for Higher Education. (ERIC Document No. 276 349)

Uhlig, G. E., & Howes, B. (1967). Attitudes toward cheating and opportunistic behavior. *Journal of Educational Research, 60,* 411–412.

Vargo, D. J. (1991) How can we deter cheating in medical school? *Journal of the American Medical Association, 266,* 2456.

Warman, E., Harvan, R. A., & Weidman, B. (1994). Dental students' attitudes toward cheating. *Journal of Dental Education, 58,* 402–405.

Weaver, K. A., Davis, S. F., Look, C., Bizzanga, V. L., & Neal, L. (1991). Examining academic dishonesty policies. *College Student Journal, 25,* 302–305.

Westerman, G. H., Grandy, T. G., Lupo, J. V., & Tamisiea, P. E. (1996). Attitudes toward cheating in dental school. *Journal of Dental Education, 60,* 285–289.

Wilhoit, S. S. (1994). Helping students avoid plagiarism. *College Teaching, 42,* 161–164.

Chapter 5

Predicting Success on the Registered Nurse Licensure Examination— 1999 Update

DONA RINALDI CARPENTER, EDD, RN
PATRICIA BAILEY, EDD, RN

INTRODUCTION

Searching for the variable or combination of variables that best predict a student's success on the registered nurse licensure examination has long been an area of research interest for nurse educators. Educators of professional nurses have a responsibility to prepare graduates capable of ensuring minimal public safety in their professional practice. The registered nurse licensure examination is one mechanism to evaluate whether students have attained minimum competency to ensure safe practice.

This literature review presents the findings of published research addressing predictors of success on the National Council Licensure Examination–Registered Nurse (NCLEX–RN) from 1976 to 1998. A brief history of licensure precedes the literature review. 67 studies published from 1976 through 1998 were included. Table 5–1 highlights the purpose, predictor variables, statistical methods, and findings for each study reviewed. For a review of literature related to predictors of success on the NCLEX–RN prior to 1976, refer to Taylor et al. (1965, 1966) and Schwirian, Baer, Basta, and Larabee (1978).

A computerized literature search was conducted using the Cumulative Index to Nursing and Allied Health Literature, First Search, Info-Track, and Allied Literature CD-ROM in addition to a manual search through indexes and references. The general topic searched was "predictors of success on the NCLEX–RN." Subtopics searched included program type (diploma, associate and baccalaureate), NCLEX–RN structure and validity, minority students, academic and nonacademic variables, and curricular issues (integration, acceleration, upper division). Dissertation Abstracts International was also used to gather data from scholarly research regarding predictors of success on NCLEX–RN. Citations were tracked from one study to another, and every attempt was made to ensure a comprehensive review.

HISTORICAL SUMMARY OF LICENSURE EXAMINATION DEVELOPMENT

The examination to become licensed as a registered nurse has evolved and changed over time (see Table 5–2). Changes in the organization of the exam and the method of administration reflect changes in nursing curriculum designs, nursing practice, and the influence of technology. A brief overview of the most significant changes in format and administration of the exam will place the studies in historical context while illuminating the impact of issues such as public safety and technology and the importance of these issues in terms of the examination's overall design and content.

The history of licensure was summarized by Matassarin-Jacobs (1989), who noted that prior to 1944, each state controlled its own licensure examination. In 1944, the National League for Nursing (NLN) became involved in a nationwide testing program and established a test blueprint known as the State Board Test Pool Examination (SBTPE). By the early 1950s, all states were using the exam, setting their own passing score. In the middle to late 1950s, the American Nurses

TABLE 5–1.
Chronological Summary of Predictor Variables
Examined in the Research Literature from 1976 to 1998

Author/ Date	Purpose	Sample	Predictor Variables	Statistical Methods	Findings
Bell & Martindill (1976)	Derive prediction equations for each of the five licensure examinations and cross-validate the predictors with an independent sample of students.	101 nursing students who graduated from a BSN program in Houston, Texas. Second sample of nurses from the same school who graduated a year later were used to cross-validate the prediction equations.	NLN achievement tests: medical surgical I, medical surgical II, nursing of children, obstetric nursing, psychiatric nursing.	Stepwise regression analysis, cross-validation correlations ($p < .01–.05$).	NLN test scores in nursing of children and obstetric nursing were consistently the best indicators of performance on SBE. The results suggest that nursing programs should develop and validate prediction equations to assist nurses in preparing for SBE.
Deardorff et al. (1976)	Develop and validate empirical equations for predicting SBE scores of graduates of an ADN program from performance on NLN achievement tests.	Graduates of a midwestern associate degree nursing program 1969–1974.	NLN achievement tests: medical nursing, surgical nursing, nursing practice, facts and principles, antepartum, postpartum, newborn, growth and development, sick children.	Multiple regression, correlation ($p < .05$).	For ADN students, selected sets of NLN Achievement Test scores were effective predictors of SBE scores.
Perez (1977)	Develop regression analysis equations for predicting SBE scores of applicants to the nursing major using predictor variables available at the completion of the sophomore year of a BSN program.	BSN graduates of a private liberal arts college, 1968–1977.	ACT scores, GPAs at various academic levels, GPAs for science and social science courses, and an NLN exam score.	Multiple regression analysis ($p < .01–.05$).	The discussion suggests that reading ability be investigated as a measure of potential success on SBE. The ACT social science reading score, GPA upon completion of the freshman year, and GPA for courses in prerequisite social sciences emerged as the most sensitive predictors of success.

TABLE 5–1.
Chronological Summary of Predictor Variables
Examined in the Research Literature from 1976 to 1998 (Continued)

Author/ Date	Purpose	Sample	Predictor Variables	Statistical Methods	Findings
Outtz (1979)	Establish predictors of success on SBTPE for black students.	110 black nursing students who graduated from a baccalaureate program between 1973 and 1977.	Cumulative GPA in high school and college, GPA in high school science and math courses, GPA in college science courses, SAT: verbal and math total.	Stepwise multiple regression, Pearson product moment correlation ($p < .01–.05$).	SAT scores were significantly correlated with SBTPE. Positive relationship between high school GPA and college GPA. Positive relationship between high school science and college science grades. Cumulative GPA in college via multiple regression analysis was best predictor of success.
Washburn (1980)	Discover the relationship between NLN Achievement Test scores and SBE performance.	166 graduates of a diploma degree school of nursing between 1976 and 1978.	Nursing care of patients 1, 2, 3.	Pearson product correlation ($p < .01$).	NLN Achievement Test scores had a highly significant correlation with SBTPE result. Nursing care of patients II was the best predictor of success. Obstetrics NLN achievement test was highest predictor of success on psychiatric section of SBTPE.
Melcolm & Bausell (1981)	Determine the degree to which the integrated curriculum influences licensure success.	390 baccalaureate graduates of the 1976 and 1977 classes at the University of Maryland School of Nursing.	NLN achievement scores, GPA, individual grades from nursing courses.	Simple correlation, forward stepwise multiple regression ($p < .01–.05$).	NLN achievement scores remain good predictors of success on STBPE.

TABLE 5–1.
Chronological Summary of Predictor Variables
Examined in the Research Literature from 1976 to 1998 (Continued)

Author/ Date	Purpose	Sample	Predictor Variables	Statistical Methods	Findings
St. Thomas (1982)	Analyze the relationship between the first-semester GPA and the SBE scores of Vermont College graduates with the ultimate goal of requiring a 1.75 QPI to continue in the nursing major.	108 freshmen nursing students.	Freshmen GPA, SBE scores.	Linear regression analysis and Pearson product moment ($p < .01–.05$).	Although a significant relationship exists between GPA and nursing board scores, a GPA of 1.75 failed to predict success in the SBE.
Aldag & Rose (1983)	Determine the relationship of age and ACT scores to college GPA and SBE scores.	787 persons admitted to an ADN program over a 10-year period.	Age, ACT scores, college GPA, SBE scores.	Pearson product moment ($p < .01$).	More older students passed SBE. Age and ACT scores were not correlated with GPA. Age and ACT scores were positively correlated with SBE scores.
Breyer (1984)	Assess the ability of the 1982 edition of the Comprehensive Nursing Achievement Test to predict NCLEX–RN score and to present equations that could predict NCLEX–RN score from the clinical content advisory subscores reported in the 1983 edition of the Comprehensive Nursing Achievement Test.	2,496 associate degree and diploma students.	Comprehensive Nursing Achievement Test.	Pearson product moment, multiple regression ($p < .001$).	Strong relationship between success on the Comprehensive Nursing Achievement Test and success on the NCLEX–RN.

TABLE 5–1.
Chronological Summary of Predictor Variables Examined in the Research Literature from 1976 to 1998 (Continued)

Author/ Date	Purpose	Sample	Predictor Variables	Statistical Methods	Findings
Dell & Halpin (1984)	Determine which variables best predicted program success on SBEs in a predominantly black BSN program.	456 black students attending a predominantly black baccalaureate school of nursing from 1970 to 1974.	SAT verbal scores, SAT quantitative scores, high school GPA, NLN prenursing.	Discriminate analysis ($p < .001–.05$).	Discriminant analysis showed that the measures significantly differentiated between dropouts and graduates.
Sharp (1984)	Determine whether any one of seven selected variables or a combination of predicted performance on the SBTPE.	322 graduates of the University of Tennessee between 1974 and 1979.	High school GPA, university GPA, ACT scores (English, mathematics, social studies, natural sciences, composite).	Discriminate analysis, stepwise multiple regression ($p < .0001$).	The variables selected were predictive of SBTPE performance. The strongest combination for predicting SBTPE performance was GPA, math, and natural science ACT scores.
Yocum & Scherubel (1985)	Examine student performance prior to and following admission to a BSN program in comparison with their performance on the individual sections of the SBTPE and an overall assessment of pass–fail on the SBTPE.	139 class of 1980 graduates.	Preadmission GPAs, individual course grades, cumulative GPAs for work completed following admission, race, the school from which the greatest number of prerequisite courses were completed, previous academic degrees, number of credit hours earned prior to admission.	Stepwise multiple regression, Pearson product moment correlation ($p < .001–.05$).	Junior and senior year cumulative clinical nursing theory GPA had the highest weighting for pass/fail on SBTPE. Clinical nursing theory GPA was more highly correlated with SBE performance than the clinical nursing practicum.

TABLE 5–1.
Chronological Summary of Predictor Variables
Examined in the Research Literature from 1976 to 1998 (Continued)

Author/ Date	Purpose	Sample	Predictor Variables	Statistical Methods	Findings
Quick et al. (1985)	Determine whether admission data can be used to predict success on the NCLEX–RN in a baccalaureate program.	182 students who received baccalaureate degrees in 1982, 1983, and 1984.	GPA end of freshman year, SAT verbal scores, anatomy and physiology grades.	Discriminant analysis ($p < .0001$).	Data available at the time of admission to the first clinical nursing course permit prediction of NCLEX–RN performance.
Felts (1986)	Determine which cognitive variables best predict success in nursing courses, and examine the relationship between selected cognitive variables and performance on the NCLEX–RN.	297 first-time writers of the NCLEX–RN between July 1992 and February 1984.	High school GPA, ACT scores, age, behavioral or social science courses, biological science courses, humanities courses, nursing courses, physical science courses, support courses, cumulative GPA.	Discriminant analysis and chi-square ($p < .001$).	ACT composite score was the best admission criteria predictor for success in nursing courses, with support course GPA and microbiology best predicting overall success in college. Performance in college courses predicted success on the NCLEX–RN with greater accuracy than high school performance. Grades in the biological and social sciences along with humanities differentiated students that pass or fail. The role of nursing courses in relation to the NCLEX–RN was not identified in this study.

TABLE 5-1.
Chronological Summary of Predictor Variables
Examined in the Research Literature from 1976 to 1998 (Continued)

Author/ Date	Purpose	Sample	Predictor Variables	Statistical Methods	Findings
Glick et al. (1986)	Investigate (a) the relationship between admission selection variables and subsequent achievement in a BSN program and on the NCLEX–RN, (b) the extent to which achievement in clinical courses predicts performance on NCLEX–RN, and (c) the relationship among predictor variables.	51 graduates, 96% female.	Admission selection variables, prenursing courses, required clinical nursing courses.	Correlation coefficients, stepwise multiple regression ($p < .001-.05$).	When GPA in nursing courses was used as criterion of success, the prenursing GPA and biology GPA correlated most highly. Statistically significant correlations observed among the predictor variables supported the validity of using academic achievement data as selection criteria for admission to a BSN program.
Payne & Duffey (1986)	Determine whether graduates of a BSN program who failed or were near failure on the NCLEX–RN could have been identified as at-risk students during their undergraduate nursing program.	144 graduates of the class of 1983 and 139 graduates of the class of 1984.	Entrance GPA, SAT math, SAT verbal, SAT total, nursing GPA.	Pearson product moment correlation and regression analysis ($p < .01-.05$).	The majority of students who are at risk of failing the NCLEX–RN can be identified fairly early in the nursing program, particularly after the first or second semester of professional study.

TABLE 5–1.
Chronological Summary of Predictor Variables
Examined in the Research Literature from 1976 to 1998 (Continued)

Author/ Date	Purpose	Sample	Predictor Variables	Statistical Methods	Findings
Whitley & Chadwick (1986)	Evaluate student curricular experience while in a BSN program following unusually low scores on the NCLEX–RN.	176 graduates of a BSN program.	SAT scores, science GPAs, cumulative GPA, school of nursing examinations.	Pearson correlation ($p < .0001–.05$).	Graduates who entered the program with low SAT scores, low cumulative and science GPAs, and scores below the class mean on school of nursing examinations were at a significantly high risk of failing the NCLEX–RN. The integrated curriculum was found to present difficulty for students.
Woodham & Taube (1986)	*Ex post facto* correlational study to determine the relationship of selected admission criteria and performance in the integrated nursing major didactic courses of an ADN program as predictors for performance on the NCLEX–RN.	104 ADN graduates.	7 required ADN courses, SAT verbal scores, age at graduation, high school class rank, SAT math scores.	Pearson correlation, multivariate regression ($p < .01$).	A significant positive relationship was demonstrated with the seven nursing courses and SAT verbal scores. Age at graduation, high school class rank, and SAT math scores were not significant in predicting NCLEX–RN performance.
Bauwens & Gerhard (1987)	To investigate the Watson–Glaser Critical Thinking Appraisal as a potential predictor of success on NCLEX–RN.	177 BSN students who graduated between December 1982 and May 1984.	University GPA/ Watson–Glaser.	Pearson product moment and stepwise multiple regression ($p < .01–.005$).	Watson–Glaser is not a valid measure of specific cognitive processes underlying the nursing process. The usefulness of the Watson–Glaser Critical Thinking Appraisal is in its ability to predict nursing success on a preadmission basis.

TABLE 5–1.
Chronological Summary of Predictor Variables
Examined in the Research Literature from 1976 to 1998 (Continued)

Author/ Date	Purpose	Sample	Predictor Variables	Statistical Methods	Findings
Crane et al. (1987)	(a) To determine the validity coefficients of selected predictor variables obtained prior to admission to the program and of eight intermediate variables reflecting scores on standardized achievement tests administered at the conclusion of each of eight course sequences; (b) to ascertain validity coefficients for the same predictors and intermediate variables for each of four ethnic groups; and (c) to identify through the use of multiple-regression analyses the combination of two or three predictor variables more predictive of success.	The records of 418 graduating nursing students who had completed a diploma nursing program between 1984 and 1985.	Chronological age, anatomy GPA, physiology GPA, psychology GPA, prerequisite total GPA, California achievement tests, reading comprehension, reading total, mathematics concepts and applications, mathematics total, anatomy and physiology, normal nutrition, NLN fundamentals of drug therapy, NLN psychiatric nursing, NLN nursing the childbearing family, NLN nursing of children.	Correlation, multiple regression ($p < .001–.05$).	Senior GPA is a highly valid predictor of NCLEX–RN scores for members of the white and Hispanic subgroups but only modestly valid for black and Asian subgroups. High school GPA affords little if any predictive validity of either criterion measure for any ethnic group. Prerequisite coursework taken primarily in a community college affords moderate predictive validity for white, Hispanic, and Asian subgroups but high validity for the black subgroup, in the prediction of senior GPA but reduced if not marginal validity for all ethnic groups. Standardized achievement tests in reading and mathematics provide somewhat mixed validity across all subgroups for both criterions measured.

TABLE 5–1.
Chronological Summary of Predictor Variables
Examined in the Research Literature from 1976 to 1998 (Continued)

Author/ Date	Purpose	Sample	Predictor Variables	Statistical Methods	Findings
Gross et al. (1987)	To evaluate the impact of the nursing curriculum on the students' ability to think critically, and to examine the relationship of performance on the Watson–Glaser Critical Thinking Appraisal and the NLN preadmission test, to GPA and NCLEX–RN.	108 associate and baccalaureate students.	Age, years of school after high school, ethnicity, Watson–Glaser at entry, Watson–Glaser at exit.	Correlations, multiple regression ($p < .01–.05$).	Nursing education improves critical thinking skills, and the GPA is more important than the Watson–Glaser in predicting NCLEX–RN performance.
Yang et al. (1987)	Investigate (a) the relationship between admission selection variables and subsequent achievement in an integrated BSN program and performance on the NCLEX–RN, (b) the extent to which achievement in clinical nursing courses predicted performance on the NCLEX–RN, and (c) the relationship among predictor variables.	210 graduates of a BSN program who graduated in 1983, 1984, and 1985.	High school record, cumulative nursing GPA, individual and composite ACT scores, grades from all required prenursing and clinical nursing courses, cumulative GPA for chemistry, biology, and microbiology.	Pearson product moment correlation, stepwise multiple regression ($p < .01–.05$).	When prenursing GPA was selected as the criterion of success, prenursing GPA and biology GPA exhibited the highest correlation coefficients among other predictors for all nursing courses. Although there were high correlations among criterion variables and NCLEX–RN scores, none of the predictors showing high correlations were significant predictors of performance on NCLEX–RN. One nursing course (Nursing III) made a significant contribution to the NCLEX scores over and above all other clinical courses.

TABLE 5–1.
Chronological Summary of Predictor Variables
Examined in the Research Literature from 1976 to 1998 (Continued)

Author/ Date	Purpose	Sample	Predictor Variables	Statistical Methods	Findings
Friedemann & Valentine (1988)	Explore prenursing student factors and their relationship to success in the licensure examination.	164 graduates from 1978 to 1984 taking the old state board exam, and 159 taking the new examination.	Age, number of academic credits completed prior to entering nursing, entry GPA, grades in inorganic or organic chemistry, grades in the program courses consisting of six nursing courses, nutrition, and pharmacology, exit GPA.	ANOVA, stepwise multiple regression ($p < .001–.05$).	GPA and student age were most useful in predicting exam scores from the preadmission variables. Students who received A grades in lecture courses scored relatively higher and B students scored lower on the new licensure examination compared to the old examinations. Students entering the program as LPNs did markedly better on the new licensure examination than on the old examinations.
Krupa et al. (1988)	Determine whether grades in nursing courses required of all students could predict NCLEX–RN performance.	The records of 384 nursing students who graduated from a BSN program and took the NCLEX–RN from 1982 through 1985.	Introduction to the process of nursing, nursing of the adult: adapting to health stressors I and II, nursing of the childbearing and childrearing family and practicum, family and community health nursing and practicum, nursing leadership and practicum, issues in nursing, research in nursing, mental health nursing in the community and practicum.	Chi-square, structured coefficient.	Grades in an introductory nursing course taken during the sophomore year and in a medical–surgical nursing course taken during the junior year were substantially and directly related to NCLEX–RN performance. Grades earned in all other nursing theory courses had positive correlations with the discriminant function. Grades in the practicum courses were relatively poor predictors of NCLEX–RN performance.

TABLE 5–1.
Chronological Summary of Predictor Variables
Examined in the Research Literature from 1976 to 1998 (Continued)

Author/ Date	Purpose	Sample	Predictor Variables	Statistical Methods	Findings
McKinney et al. (1988)	Determine which measures of academic success predicted success on the NCLEX–RN.	136 BSN students from a private liberal arts college between 1983 and 1985.	SAT total, SAT math, SAT verbal, GPA, Mosby Assess Test scores, age, sex, courses repeated, Type A behavior.	Multiple regression and Pearson product moment ($p < .01-.001$).	Nurse educators could identify students early in programs whose academic patterns suggest potential difficulty within the nursing major and likely failure on the NCLEX–RN.
Feldt & Donahue (1989)	Identify the best linear combination of readily available scholastic variables, one set to predict success in a nursing program and the other to predict performance on the NCLEX–RN.	155 students who completed and 34 who failed to complete a BSN program for 1984–1986.	GPA, ACT composite score, chemistry grade, anatomy grade, high school percentile rank.	Multiple regression, Chi-square, correlation ($p < .001$).	The best set of predictors of nursing GPA included ACT composite score, anatomy grade, and chemistry grade. The best set of predictors of NCLEX–RN included ACT composite score, high school percentile rank, nursing GPA, and chemistry grade.
Jenks et al. (1989)	Identify predictors of success in the NCLEX–RN and determine the optimal time to identify students at risk.	407 graduates of an integrated upper division BSN program from 1984 to 1987.	Lower division GPA, science GPA, type of lower division college, age, sex, junior-level nursing course grades, senior-level nursing grades, Mosby Assess Test.	Pearson correlation coefficient, stepwise regression analysis ($p < .0001-.01$).	Students at high risk can be identified at the end of the junior year so that enrichment and support programs can be introduced at that time.

TABLE 5–1.
Chronological Summary of Predictor Variables
Examined in the Research Literature from 1976 to 1998 (Continued)

Author/ Date	Purpose	Sample	Predictor Variables	Statistical Methods	Findings
Dell & Valine (1990)	Determine multivariate relationships among collegiate GPA, SAT/ACT scores, self-esteem, and age in explaining differences in scores on the NCLEX–RN made by new graduates of BSN programs.	90 senior generic nursing students in three small, 4-year public southeastern schools of nursing.	GPA, SAT/ACT Z scores, self-esteem measures, age.	Spearman-Brown correlation, multiple regression ($p < .001$).	GPA is one of the best predictors of success on national nursing examinations. There was a lack of contribution to the variance by the self-esteem measures.
Lengacher (1990)	Examine the relationship between selected admission variables, age, perception or role strain, achievement in clinical and nursing courses, achievement on NLN examinations, exit GPA, and performance on NCLEX–RN examination.	146 associate degree graduates.	Entrance GPA, ACT subtest scores, age, perception of role strain, achievement in clinical and nursing courses, achievement on NLN examinations, exit GPA.	Correlation coefficients, stepwise multiple regression ($p < .001–.05$).	The best predictor of performance on the NCLEX–RN of the selected admission variables were exit GPA and ACT composite scores. Nurse educators can identify students early in the program who would be successful on the NCLEX–RN and those who would be at risk for failure.

TABLE 5.1.
Chronological Summary of Predictor Variables
Examined in the Research Literature from 1976 to 1998 (Continued)

Author/ Date	Purpose	Sample	Predictor Variables	Statistical Methods	Findings
Foti & DeYoung (1991)	Retrospective correlational study to determine variables that predict success on the NCLEX–RX.	296 nursing students who graduated between 1985 and 1988.	GPA, overall GPA in major, GPA in science, SAT verbal and quantitative, NLN Baccalaureate Achievement Test score, Mosby Assess Test score.	Pearson correlation and multiple regression analysis ($p < .0001$).	Pearson correlations indicated the Mosby Assess Test, overall GPA, GPA in the major, NLN Achievement Test, and SAT verbal to be of moderate predictive value. Multiple regression analysis indicated that the most useful combination of predictors was the Mosby Assess Test, SAT verbal, and overall GPA.
Horns et al. (1991)	Determine predictors of success on the NCLEX preadmission and years 2, 3, and 4 variables in relation to NCLEX–RN scores.	408 BSN students.	Age, sex, race, admission GPA, grades for clinical courses, grades for clinical courses in mental health, adult health, and maternal child nursing, senior clinical course grades, NLN comprehensive exam, graduate GPA.	Forward regression analysis, correlation coefficients ($p < .01$).	Preadmission and sophomore year predictors of NCLEX–RN success could be used to design early interventions for students performing poorly and at risk of failing the NCLEX–RN.
Poorman & Martin (1991)	Determine the relationship of test anxiety, cognition, and general academic performance of second-semester senior-level BSN students to success on the NCLEX–RN.	102 senior BSN students.	Test anxiety inventory, cognitive assessment tool, quality point average, SAT scores.	Multiple regression, Pearson product moment correlation, chi-square ($p < .05$).	Test anxiety was inversely related to passing score on the NCLEX–RN. Academic aptitude positively correlated with passing scores on the NCLEX–RN. Negative cognition was not inversely related to pass rate on the NCLEX–RN. Self-perceived grades and self-predicted NCLEX–RN scores were the best predictors of actual NCLEX–RN scores. Subjects successful on the NCLEX–RN were more likely to believe they were good test-takers and reported more facilitative thoughts during exams than those who failed the NCLEX–RN.

TABLE 5–1.
Chronological Summary of Predictor Variables
Examined in the Research Literature from 1976 to 1998 (Continued)

Author/ Date	Purpose	Sample	Predictor Variables	Statistical Methods	Findings
Fowles (1992)	Identify predictors of success on the NCLEX–RN and within the nursing curriculum.	192 graduates of an upper division, single-purpose BSN program.	GPA, ACT composite, A & P grades, Mosby Assess Test.	Stepwise multiple regression analysis, correlation coefficients ($p < .05$).	NCLEX–RN success can be predicted, and findings have implications for entering a nursing student into an early intervention program.
Mills et al. (1992)	Identify academic predictors of success on the NCLEX–RN for nurse candidates who graduated from a 4-year BSN program and to describe the odds for success of nurse candidates on their first attempt at the NCLEX–RN.	534 first-time nurse candidates.	Age, sex, high school GPA, four subscores (social science, natural science, mathematics, and English), transfer, cumulative GPA for nursing courses at the end of each of the 4 academic years.	Stepwise logistic regression ($p < .05$).	Cumulative GPA suggested that the end of the sophomore year was the best time for predicting success and the end of the junior year was best for predicting failure. Age was inversely related to successful performance in three of the four models.
Mills et al. (1992)	Identify predictors of successful performance and determine probabilities of success on the NCLEX–RN.	328 first-time nurse candidates for the NCLEX–RN from 1982 to 1990.	Age, sex, education, GPA, graduate work, cumulative semester GPA.	Logistic regression ($p < .05$).	The best time for predicting NCLEX–RN performance is at the end of an accelerated program.

TABLE 5–1.
Chronological Summary of Predictor Variables Examined in the Research Literature from 1976 to 1998 (Continued)

Author/ Date	Purpose	Sample	Predictor Variables	Statistical Methods	Findings
McClelland et al. (1992)	Validate, using a statewide sample, findings from two previous smaller investigations on the relationships between admission selection variables and subsequent achievement in BSN programs and performance on the NCLEX–RN.	1,069 graduates of nine Iowa basic baccalaureate programs.	Relationship between admission selection variables and subsequent achievement in the nursing program; the extent to which achievement in nursing courses predicted performance on the NCLEX–RN. Path analysis was used to formulate a causal model describing the relationships among the variables in the study.	Pearson product moment correlation coefficients, stepwise multiple regression ($p < .001–.01$).	Prenursing GPA and ACT scores predict performance on the NCLEX–RN.
Rami (1992)	Evaluate the importance of four predictor variables in predicting success on the NCLEX–RN.	35 graduates of a newly developed BSN program.	Prenursing GPA, ACT scores, comprehensive examination, Basics I NLN Achievement Test.	Multiple regression analysis, Pearson product moment ($p < .001–.05$).	Findings according to author were inconclusive. Basic I test scores were significantly correlated with success on the NCLEX–RN and were significant predictors of success. The author recommended repeating the study with a larger sample.
Younger & Grap (1992)	Identify the best risk indices for students who do not pass NCLEX–RN, pinpoint the earliest time in their academic careers that their risk can substantially be known, and estimate the effectiveness of a formal review course.	388 graduates of an upper division BSN who took the NCLEX–RN examination between 1984 and 1987.	Nursing school course grades, SAT scores, NLN test scores.	Correlation, stepwise multiple regression.	Nursing course grades, SAT scores, and NLN test scores can be used in combination to predict NCLEX–RN performance. Whether a student took an NCLEX–RN review course was not a significant predictor of performance.

TABLE 5–1.
Chronological Summary of Predictor Variables
Examined in the Research Literature from 1976 to 1998 (Continued)

Author/ Date	Purpose	Sample	Predictor Variables	Statistical Methods	Findings
Friarson et al. (1993)	Assess the associated effects of a three-pronged intervention procedure on NCLEX–RN performance.	8 African–American nursing students.	The three-pronged approach consisted of instructions in effective test-taking, participation in learning teams, follow-up activities conducted by the faculty to reinforce the first two components.	Correlation ($p < .025$).	The three-pronged intervention effort significantly improved NCLEX–RN passing rate and mean score.
Wall et al. (1993)	Identify academic variables both before and during the nursing program that predict success or failure on NCLEX–RN and to determine how accurately students at risk of failure can be identified.	92 graduates of an NLN-accredited BSN program in a private, church-affiliated liberal arts college in the Midwest.	SAT, high school rank, NLN tests, Mosby Assess Test.	t-test, discriminant function analysis ($p < .01$–$.15$).	Data collected prior to entry in nursing program can be used to predict performance on current NCLEX–RN. Several variables were significantly better performance predictors: high school rank, sophomore GPA, GPA in sciences, nursing and senior GPA, and NLN achievement tests taken at end of each nursing course.
Waterhouse et al. (1993)	Identify variables that might be used as predictors for success on the post-1988 NCLEX–RN and to identify those students at risk of failing the examination.	257 graduates of a BSN program from 1988 to 1990.	15 variables examined, SAT verbal, SAT math, high school percentile, physiology grade, pathophysiology grade, second junior nursing course grade, first senior nursing course grade, sophomore GPI, graduation GPI, last nursing clinical.	Pearson product moment correlation coefficients ($p < .05$).	Reasonably accurate predictive data on individual students' performance are available by the end of the junior year, allowing faculty to begin interventions for at-risk students.

TABLE 5–1.
Chronological Summary of Predictor Variables Examined in the Research Literature from 1976 to 1998 (Continued)

Author/Date	Purpose	Sample	Predictor Variables	Statistical Methods	Findings
Heupel (1994)	Examine the relationship of selected academic variables to NCLEX–RN performance and determine a "best set" of indicators predictive of NCLEX–RN success.	152 basic students who completed the BSN program between 1985 and 1987.	Freshman GPA, sophomore GPA, junior GPA, senior GPA, theory grades for five prerequisite science courses, theory grades for three sophomore medical-surgical nursing courses, theory grades for six junior medical–surgical and parent–child nursing courses, theory grades for four senior mental health, community health, and leadership nursing courses.	Multiple regression analysis and Pearson product moment correlation coefficients ($p < .0001–.05$).	The best predictors were a sophomore nursing theory course, a junior nursing theory course, the junior year GPA, and a senior nursing theory course. Selected nursing theory courses and the junior GPA could be used in a statistical model to predict success on the NCLEX–RN.
Drake & Michael (1995)	Establish criterion-related validity for selected measures used to predict passing or failing on the NCLEX–RN.	350 ADN students.	Theory grades for eight nursing theory courses, six nursing laboratory courses, four biology-related courses, GPA prior to admission.	Predictive validity coefficients and factor analysis.	The most valid predictor was GPA in the eight nursing theory courses.
Alexander & Brophy (1997)	Identify admission, progression, and exit variables that predict performance on NCLEX–RN and determine those variables that identify students at risk.	Quota sample of 188 ADN graduates.	High school rank, SAT scores, years of high school chemistry and math, admission status, GPA, age, theory courses, NLN Comprehensive Achievement Test.	t-tests, chi-square, logistic regression.	The strongest indicators of success were SAT verbal scores, nursing GPA, and NLN Comprehensive Achievement Test scores.

TABLE 5–1.
Chronological Summary of Predictor Variables
Examined in the Research Literature from 1976 to 1998 (Continued)

Author/ Date	Purpose	Sample	Predictor Variables	Statistical Methods	Findings
Arathuzik & Aber (1998)	Identify academic and nonacademic factors associated with NCLEX–RN success in nursing students enrolled in a public college of nursing with a diverse student population.	79 generic senior students.	Four tools used: demographic data sheet, the Internal Block Scale, the External Block Scale, and the Study Skills Self-Efficacy Instrument.	Descriptive statistics.	Several internal and external blocks to success were described by students, including family responsibilities, emotional distress, fatigue, and financial and work burdens. Significant correlations were found between success in the NCLEX–RN and cumulative undergraduate nursing program GPA, English as the primary language spoken at home, lack of family responsibilities or demands, lack of emotional distress, and sense of competency in critical thinking.

ACT = American College Testing exam
ASN = associate degree in nursing
ANOVA = analysis of variance
BSN = bachelor of science–nursing
GPA = grade point average
LPN = licensed practical nurse
NCLEX–RN = National Council Licensure Examination–Registered Nurse
NLN = National League for Nursing
QPI = Quality Product Index
SAT = Scholastic Aptitude Test
SBE = State Board Examination
SBTPE = State Board Test Pool Examination

TABLE 5–2.
Historical Evolution and Characteristics of the Licensure Examination

Examination Title	Date of Inception	Number of Questions	Format	Passing Score
State Board Test Pool Examination	1944	600	Five content areas: medical, surgical, pediatrics, obstetrics, psychiatric	350 minimum for each content area
National Council Licensure Examination	1982	400	Integrated, eight areas of human functioning, nursing process, and locus of control	1,600
National Council Licensure Examination	1988	300	Integrated, four areas of client needs, nursing process	Pass/fail
Computerized Adaptive Testing Licensure Examination	1994	50–300	Integrated, four areas of client needs, nursing process; completed at the computer	Pass/fail

Association, became involved in control of the examination while the NLN continued to administer it.

The National Council of State Boards of Nursing (NCSBN) assumed responsibility for licensure test development and administration in 1978 and continues to maintain this responsibility. A five-part, content-based examination was initially developed with a passing score set yearly. A normative reference format was used (Matassarin-Jacobs, 1989).

In 1982, the examination was redesigned from normative referencing to criterion referencing and from a five-part format to a unified integrated test. The focus of the integration was the nursing process and included eight areas of human functioning. The overall passing score was set at 1600 (Matassarin-Jacobs, 1989). After July 1988 the examination scoring was changed to pass/fail. Nursing process continued to be the basis for the overall design of the examination in addition to four areas of client needs: safety, physiological integrity, psychosocial integrity, and health promotion. The examination continues to be criterion referenced (Matassarin-Jacobs, 1989).

Scoring changes to pass/fail had far-reaching effects. According to Washburn and Short (1992), student preparation for and performance on the pass/fail examination were affected by these scoring changes. In Washburn and Short's study, nursing education administrators were surveyed regarding their "knowledge of NCLEX–RN changes, their opinions regarding the changes, and their involvement in the change process" (p. 17). Approximately three fourths of the administrators—75.8% bachelor of science nursing programs (BSN) and 71.4% associate degree nursing programs (ADN)—reported that they were not well informed (p. 172).

The original random study sample included 100 administrators of BSN programs and 100 administrators of ADN programs for a total of 200. The response rate was 60% ($N = 120$) with approximately half of the respondents from the BSN program and half from the ADN degree program. The tool had been pilot tested using 10 nursing program administrators randomly selected from BSN and ADN programs and was reviewed for content validity and clarity. Since the overall response rate was above 50% on the mailed questionnaire and the sample was randomly chosen, one can have confidence in the validity of these findings.

Bosma (1992), executive director of the NCSBN, responded to the research reported by Washburn and Short (1992) in a letter to the editor. She emphasized strategies used by the national council for decisions regarding content coverage and the setting of passing standards that are valid and fair.

According to the NCSBN (1990), difficulty of test items and the number of test items had no effect on the passing rate. This is because the passing standards on the NCLEX–RN are criterion referenced, which means "the standard is referenced to the content and difficulty of test items, as opposed to a norm-referenced approach, in which the standard is referenced to the performance of a normative group of examinees" (NCSBN, 1990, p. 10). A change in the passing standard will effect a change in the passing rate unless the level of candidate competence (ability to practice entry-level nursing safely and effectively as measured by the NCLEX–RN) changes. "Effective with the July 1988 examination, the RN passing standard was increased slightly, so that candidates had to answer approximately three more items correctly in order to pass the examination. This increase, and a simultaneous drop in the NCLEX-estimated competence level of candidates taking the July 1988 examination was associated with a drop in the passing rate of approximately eight percentage points" (Matassarin-Jacobs, 1989, p. 12).

In the late 1980s, the NCSBN devoted considerable time, money, and effort to develop computerized adaptive testing (CAT). Field tests for CAT were conducted in July 1990 and February 1991. The purpose was to determine the feasibility of using a CAT mode for administering licensure tests by studying the efficiency, measurement properties, logistics, and costs. Analysis of the data from these field trials showed that CAT measured candidates' performance in a manner comparable with the previous paper-and-pencil type of administration. It was also determined that neither demographics nor prior computer experience had any effect on performance. In addition, the CAT was determined to be psychometrically sound (NCSBN, 1993, p. 11). CAT is based on the principle that for each examinee, some questions will be more effective than others in revealing levels of competence. As the candidate answers each question, the computer calculates a competence level.

National implementation of this examination method, which is based on a psychometric model known as item response theory (IRT), was initiated by NCSBN in July 1994. "The central concept of IRT is the item characteristic curve (ICC), a function that represents the probability of answering a given item correctly given an examinee's latent trait or ability. It is assumed that as ability increases, so does the probability of answering an item correctly" (Halkitis & Leahy, 1993, p. 380).

This method of testing presents both students and faculty with new challenges for the teaching–learning process. These challenges include ensuring that students are comfortable using computerized testing and developing critical thinking skills that promote sound decision making and problem solving in clinical situations. The student will benefit from the test's being structured for the individual and administered more frequently. Other benefits are that the test will not pass marginal candidates, thus improving protection of the public, it will lessen or eliminate the need for temporary permits, and it will help alleviate supply problems by providing more immediate results, thus putting new nurses in the mainstream of the workplace more quickly (NCSBN, 1989).

A step into future technology has been taken by the NCSBN in its work toward a computerized clinical simulation test (CST) of nursing competence. The intent of this project is to address performance assessment concerns that paper-and-pencil examinations are not capable of evaluating. Competence to practice professional nursing would be better evaluated using a simulated type testing procedure that requires decision-making and problem-solving skills. Based on the nursing process, the examinee is given a case study and then must proceed with data gathering and intervention activities (NCSBN, 1993, p. 1). The client responds to these activities as the examinee moves through the simulation. Study of this project was to be conducted through 1997 Bersky, Krawczak, and Kuma (1998) described "how CST works, the case development and scoring key development processes, and the plans for the CST pilot study scheduled for spring 1998" (p. 20). "In August 1999, based on a report of the study findings, the National Council's Delegate Assemble (voting membership) will make a decision regarding the use of CST as a component of the NCLEX–RN examination" (Bersky et al., 1998, p. 25).

THE LICENSURE EXAMINATION: HOW VALID IS IT?

The purpose of licensure is to ensure that professional nursing provides competent, safe nursing care to the public. The licensure examination is currently our only measurement for minimum safe practice and therefore must be a valid and reliable measure of the knowledge required to practice professional nursing.

Kane (1982) further addressed issues of validity on professional licensure examinations as well as issues surrounding content validity and how this might be ascertained. One suggestion included having a committee of experienced practitioners or "experts" decide which nursing competencies need to be evaluated.

Kane (1982) suggested that using direct observation and/or asking practitioners how they spend their working hours are two ways to determine what goes on in practice, providing data on the kinds of demands placed on practitioners. "The major difficulty with studies of how professionals spend their time is that many of the activities that appear in the results of the studies may not involve service to clients, and therefore may not be closely related to the purpose of licensure—protection of the public" (Kane, 1982, p. 912). Questioning the validity of licensure examinations is critical if we are to do what we promise with the exam—ensure public safety. The CST, should it be incorporated into the licensure exam, would address the concerns expressed by Kane.

Froman and Owen (1989) questioned the validity of the change in licensure examination from the State Board Examination (SBE) to that developed by the NCSBN (NCLEX–RN). Although the emphasis on the nursing process as the model of care seemed appropriate for testing, the authors cited the sparsity of evidence in regard to concurrent, predictive, or construct validity for both the SBE and the NCLEX–RN (p. 334). Also to be considered is that the licensure examination still does not differentiate between diploma, associate, and baccalaureate degree programs.

According to the NCSBN (1993), job analysis is an essential first step in the development of NCLEX–RN. "The validity of a licensure examination (such as NCLEX) rests squarely on the relationship of the examination to safe and effective practice. The primary focus of the relationship to practice is the examination's job analysis based on content validity. NCLEX administered by CAT is clearly valid from this perspective" (NCSBN, 1993, p. 6).

Job analysis is conducted every three years and involves collecting data on nursing activities performed by a stratified random sample of over 3,000 newly licensed nurses. Nursing activities are rated regarding frequency and criticality of each activity. The data are submitted to statistical testing, and, along with expert judgment, the test plan is reviewed and revised. Item development is then implemented through NCLEX–RN development panels. Item writers are selected, trained, and assisted in developing the examination. The minimum standard or passing point is reviewed by a panel of judges every three years. Changes in the passing point are made as necessary (Campbell-Warnock, Jones-Dickson, & Fields, 1993).

PREDICTORS OF SUCCESS IN BACCALAUREATE, ASSOCIATE, AND DIPLOMA NURSING PROGRAMS

Predicting success on the NCLEX–RN has always been a concern of nurse educators in baccalaureate, associate, and diploma programs. Predictors are those factors that provide the best measure of a student's ability to succeed on the licensure examination. Some predictors may be very program specific, such as grades in science courses or nursing courses. Other predictors are more standardized measures such as NLN Achievement Tests and the Mosby Assess Test. Each program must evaluate individually the variables that will best predict their graduates' success on the licensure examination. The following review emphasizes variables that have had the most predictive value for baccalaureate, associate, and diploma programs and that can provide direction for others initiating such studies.

Baccalaureate Programs

A number of research studies addressing predictors of success in baccalaureate nursing programs have focused on preadmission criteria as indicators of success on the NCLEX–RN. High school grade-point average (GPA) and subscales of the American College Testing Exam (ACT) are two predictor variables that have been used in numerous studies. Mills, Sampel, Pohlman, and Becker (1992), in their study of 534 nurse candidates for the NCLEX–RN from 1982 to 1990, used stepwise logistic regression as the multivariate technique and found the admission variables of GPA and ACT scores to be weak predictors of examination performance. Logistic regression was appropriate since it requires neither the assumption of a normal distribution for NCLEX–RN pass rates nor the multivariate normality of GPA and ACT scores. However, several studies found the admission GPA to be useful in predicting successful performance on the NCLEX–RN (Friedemann & Valentine, 1988; Horns, O'Sullivan, & Goodman, 1991; Payne & Duffy, 1986; Sharp, 1984; Stronck, 1979; Yocom & Scherubel, 1985). All of the previous authors used stepwise multiple regression in their analysis of admission GPA and performance on NCLEX–RN except for Horns et al. (1991), who used a forward regression procedure. Given that the same model for regression was used in the majority of the referenced studies, the results are more reliable in predicting NCLEX–RN success. GPA and ACT scores appear to be valid variables to predict success on the NCLEX–RN at the completion of a baccalaureate nursing program.

Yang, Glick, and McClelland (1987) included high school rank as a variable and found a direct correlation with NCLEX–RN scores and ACT social science subscores. Scholastic Aptitude Test (SAT) and ACT subscale scores have also been investigated as predictors of performance on the NCLEX–RN. Some studies have found the verbal and social science scores to be high predictors of performance (Foti & DeYoung, 1991; McClelland, Yang, & Glick, 1992; McKinney, Small, O'Dell, & Coonrod, 1988; Payne & Duffey, 1986; Perez, 1977; Quick, Krupa, & Whitley, 1985; Sharp, 1984; Whitley & Chadwick, 1986; Yang et al., 1987). However, Dell and Valine (1990) found "the SAT/ACT scores added nothing significant to the explanation of the variance of the NCLEX–RN scores beyond that of GPA" (p. 161). In this study both GPA and SAT/ACT scores were highly correlated, which resulted in the finding that SAT/ACT scores did not significantly add to the variance of the NCLEX–RN scores beyond that of the GPA.

A number of studies included variations of the GPA as predictors of NCLEX–RN success. Sharp (1984), Payne and Duffey (1986), and Glick, McClelland, and Yang (1986) found that math and natural science GPAs had predictive value. Cumulative GPAs at various points throughout the four years of a baccalaureate program were found to strengthen prediction for passing the licensure examination (Foti & DeYoung, 1991; Horns et al., 1991; Mills, Becker, Sampel, & Pohlman, 1992; Mills et al., 1992; St. Thomas, 1982). Marquis and Worth (1992) used descriptive statistics and Pearson correlation coefficients as well as varimax rotated factor analysis. These authors reported nursing GPA, nonnursing GPA, and faculty clinical evaluations (Like scale grading 1 = *poor* and 5 = *superior*) of students during their eight clinical rotations to be correlated with passing NCLEX–RN scores. The authors found these three factors to be closely related, although the nursing GPA and nonnursing GPA most closely defined the predictive factor.

There are a variety of factors to consider when examining GPA and specific courses in terms of their value in predicting success on the NCLEX–RN. Although each baccalaureate program has similar goals, specific coursework in general education and nursing will vary. These variations will no doubt influence their value as predictors of NCLEX–RN success; therefore, each program must evaluate these variables individually. They will not have the same predictive value for all baccalaureate programs.

The NLN test scores were used as predictors in numerous studies. Bell and Martindill (1976) found the NLN scores for Nursing of Children and Obstetric Nursing to be indicators of SBE success, and Melcolm and Bausell (1981) reported that all NLN Achievement Tests had predictive value. Foti and DeYoung (1991) and Younger and Grap (1992) reported the NLN Baccalaureate Achievement Test to have a high correlation with NCLEX–RN success. Rami (1992) found that NLN Basic I Test Scores correlated with NCLEX–RN success.

More recent studies have used the Mosby Assess Test as a predictor of NCLEX–RN and have reported positive correlations (Foti & DeYoung, 1991; Jenks, Selekman, Bross, & Paquet, 1989; and McKinney et al., 1988). The NLN Achievement Tests and Mosby Assess Test are standardized examinations and are therefore more consistent and reliable in predicting success on the

NCLEX–RN. Using Pearson correlations and multiple regression techniques in the NLN examinations and Mosby Assess Test studies, researchers have consistently evaluated these methods as positive predictors of NCLEX–RN success.

Ashley (1990) studied the effects of three NCLEX–RN preparation programs on nursing knowledge test anxiety and licensure examination performance. All subjects achieved high scores on a nursing achievement test and showed slight reduction in overall test anxiety. No statistical differences were found for the NCLEX–RN passing rates of the three groups.

Sheil and Meisenheimer (1992) reported a research study using a two-day anxiety-reducing workshop with a mixed group of new graduates in an acute care setting. All subjects experienced a reduction in anxiety as measured by Zung's Self-Rating Anxiety Scale and all participants passed the NCLEX–RN examination.

Studies addressing test anxiety are important since test anxiety can be an important factor in students' ability to succeed on the examination. Identifying test anxiety early in the students' academic careers can offer an opportunity to master test-taking skills while at the same time mastering content.

Zink (1991) conducted a retrospective study of 236 baccalaureate graduates from a single university and found the following:

1. Prenursing GPA is a good predictor of success on the NCLEX–RN.
2. Science course GPAs are positively correlated with performance on the NCLEX–RN.
3. Students' cumulative nursing course GPAs show a positive correlation with NCLEX–RN performance.
4. Nursing courses in the junior and senior year show a direct correlation with performance on the NCLEX–RN (p. 64–65).

A study of 384 graduates of a BSN program who took the NCLEX–RN from 1982 to 1985 was conducted by Krupa, Quick, and Whitley (1988). Grades for an introductory nursing course and a junior-level nursing course were found to be related to successful NCLEX–RN performance. The investigators concluded, "Grades in nursing courses hold a great deal of promise as predictors of performance on the NCLEX–RN" (p. 297). Friedemann and Valentine (1988) also found nursing lecture course grades to be better predictors of NCLEX success than clinical courses. In addition, Younger and Grap (1992) found nursing school course grades in combination with SAT scores and NLN test scores to predict NCLEX–RN success. Heupel's study (1994) of 152 baccalaureate students described the best predictors of NCLEX–RN success to be a sophomore and junior nursing theory course, the junior year GPA, and a senior nursing theory course.

Waterhouse, Carroll, & Beeman (1993), in a study of 257 graduates from one program during the years 1988 to 1990, found the two best predictors of NCLEX–RN success to be the first senior-level nursing course grade and the graduation grade point index. In addition, accurate prediction data were compiled on 86% of the students by the end of their junior year of study, and this gradually increased to 91% by the time of graduation.

Results on the latest NCLEX–RN initiated in 1988 were studied by Wall, Miller, and Widerquist (1993). Findings suggested similarities regarding predictors among this latest NCLEX–RN (pass/fail score) and the prior one (numerical score). The high school rank, prenursing science GPA, and sophomore GPA were found to be positive predictors. In addition, NLN Achievement Test scores, nursing GPA, and the Mosby Assess Test score were significant predictors of NCLEX–RN performance for this group of 92 graduates from the 1988–1991 classes of a BSN program.

Nonacademic variables have also been found to affect NCLEX–RN success rates. Poorman and Martin (1991) reported test anxiety to be inversely related to passing scores on NCLEX–RN and the "best predictors of actual NCLEX performance were self-predicted NCLEX scores and self- perceived grades [not actual GPA but the letter grade that the students believed best described their performance]" (p. 30). Ashley and O'Neil (1991) described a long-term intervention program consisting of test coaching and test-taking skills to be effective for at-risk students in passing the NCLEX–RN.

Barkley, Rhodes, and Dufour (1998) reported on the use of the NCLEX–RN Risk Appraisal Instrument to predict success on the licensure examination. The authors reported a significant relationship between passing the NCLEX–RN and scores on selected NLN Achievement Tests and grades in required nursing courses. Failure risk increased with the numbers of C's earned in required nursing courses and low scores on the Adult, Obstetric, and Psychiatric NLN Achievement Tests.

Associate Degree Nursing Programs

Deardorff, Denner, and Miller (1976) studied graduates from one ADN program between the years of 1969 and 1974. Multiple regression and correlation analysis was used to compare performance on NLN Achievement Tests with scores on the SBE. The specific achievement tests of Sick Children, Medical Nursing, and Postpartum were found to predict SBE scores (p. 38). Aldag and Rose (1983) examined a sample of 787 students admitted to an ADN program over a span of 10 years. Two groups comprised the sample: 555 traditional students who were admitted based on high school rank and composite scores on the ACT or equivalent, and 232 nontraditional students admitted based on obtaining a 2.00 GPA after completing 18 semester hours in the college. All interval data were analyzed with the analysis of variance (ANOVA) and Pearson product moment techniques, and the level of significance was set at $p < .01$. Results of the study pointed to a negative age bias on the ACT. In addition, the proportion of the older students who graduate and initially pass state boards was found to be larger than the proportion of the younger group (p. 71). "No significant differences were found between the traditional and nontraditional admissions for graduation rate or initial pass rate for the state board" (p. 71). However age was "positively related to performance on the state board examinations" (p. 73) and for this sample of ADN students, the nontraditional admission criterion (2.00 GPA in an 18-hour program of study in the college instead of high school rank and ACT scores) proved to be predictive.

Woodham and Taube (1986) examined three graduating classes from an ADN degree program. Seven required nursing courses, SAT verbal and math scores, age at graduation, and high school class rank were chosen as predictor variables. All seven nursing courses and SAT verbal scores had a significant positive relationship with passing the NCLEX–RN ($p = < .01$) (p. 115). Lengacher and Keller (1990) examined multiple admission variables (entrance GPA, ACT scores in English and math, and composite ACT scores), age, perception of role strain, achievement in clinical and nursing courses, NLN examination scores, exit GPA, and performance on NCLEX–RN among 146 graduates who wrote the exam in 1987 and 1988. The best predictors were found to be the exit GPA, ACT composite scores, two nursing theory courses in the second year of the program, and the Basic Two and Psychiatric NLN examinations (p. 163). Felts (1986) reported similar findings. Data analysis of 297 first-time writers of the NCLEX–RN between 1982 and 1984 revealed that the ACT composite score was the best admission criteria predictor for success in nursing courses and that overall college performance predicted pass/fail status on the NCLEX–RN better than did high school criteria. Grades in the sciences and the humanities differentiated students who passed and failed the NCLEX–RN. Age and licensure as an LPN did not predict NCLEX–RN performance. Drake and Michael (1995) concluded that GPA in a composite of eight theory courses was most predictive of success on the NCLEX–RN in associate degree graduates.

Breyer (1984) studied a sample of 511 associate degree graduates and 350 diploma graduates and found "a strong relationship between success on the Comprehensive Nursing Achievement Test and success on the Nurse Licensure Examination" (p. 194). Cloud-Hardaway (1988) conducted an ex post facto study of 558 ADN graduates who wrote the NCLEX–RN in 1983 and 1984. Significant relationships were found among the Mosby Assess Test scores and semester averages and success on the NCLEX–RN. Alexander and Brophy (1997) noted that "the strongest indicators of success were SAT verbal scores, nursing grade point average, and NLN Comprehensive Achievement Test scores" (p. 443).

Variables examined to predict success on the licensure examination for graduates of ADN programs are similar to those used in BSN. Since ADN programs have a greater tendency to attract nontraditional students (older students, second-career students, students with families), different personality factors must be considered when attempting to predict performance on the licensure examination. For example, the fact that students may be older and may have responsibilities such as work and home must be taken into consideration.

Diploma Nursing Programs

Washburn (1980) conducted a study of 166 graduates of a diploma program between the years 1976 and 1978. She found a significant correlation between the NLN Achievement Tests (Nursing Care of Patients I, II and II; Obstetric Nursing; Psychiatric Nursing and Nursing of Children) and SBTPE results. Results of Breyer's study (1984) of 2,496 associate degree and diploma students supported the NLN Comprehensive Nursing Achievement Test as a predictor of NCLEX–RN performance.

Two studies focused on critical thinking and predictors of success in a nursing program. Gross, Takazawa, and Rose (1987) found that critical thinking as measured by the Watson–Glaser Critical Thinking Appraisal scale improved over the four years but was not predictive of NCLEX–RN success; NCLEX–RN success was best predicted by the GPA. Bauwens and Gerhard (1987) found the Watson–Glaser Critical Thinking Appraisal scale to be useful as a preadmission predictor of nursing success. Critical thinking skills are necessary to ensure sound decision making and problem solving in clinical situations. The emphasis placed on critical thinking by the NLN further supports the need for developing these skills in nursing students. The next step is to measure these skills and examine them in terms of their ability to predict success on the licensure examination.

Special Needs of Minority Students

Several researchers looked specifically at minority students and what might predict success on the NCLEX–RN. Outtz (1979) found that high school GPA correlated with college GPA and that SAT scores were highly correlated with SBTPE scores. The cumulative college GPA was the best predictor and the SAT verbal component was the second best predictor of success on the license examination. Dell and Halpin (1984) found the senior year GPA, SAT verbal component, and the NLN prenursing test to be the best predictors of success. Boyle (1986) compared two minority groups, blacks and nonblacks, and discovered the entering GPA and ACT scores to be the best predictors of success, with ACT the strongest and best predictor. Crane, Wright, and Michael (1987) studied predictor variables for 418 minority students seeking a diploma in nursing; the subject group included Hispanic, black, Asian, and white students. For the white and Hispanic groups, the GPA for nursing courses was the most valid predictor of NCLEX–RN success, and selected NLN Achievement Tests gave higher predictive validity for the black and Asian groups. Students who took courses at a community college prior to entering the program tended to achieve higher GPAs in their nursing courses, but there was little predictive validity for the NCLEX–RN based on this variable. The NLN Achievement Tests proved to be positive predictors for both nursing course GPA and success on NCLEX–RN. Wells (1991) examined issues surrounding international predictive testing and emphasized the need to ensure that foreign-educated nurses are prepared comparably to their U.S. peers and are reasonably prepared to take a predictive exam.

Endres (1997), in a study of African-American and foreign-born baccalaureate graduates, found that "students with a Mosby Assess Test percentile rank below 21 and a D or F in a nursing course were more likely to fail the NCLEX–RN than those with a higher percentile rank and no Ds or Fs" (p. 365).

Arathuzik and Aber (1998) examined "academic and nonacademic factors associated with NCLEX–RN success in nursing students enrolled in a public college of nursing with a diverse student population" (p. 119). According to the authors,

> Significant correlations were found between success in the NCLEX–RN and cumulative undergraduate nursing program grade point average, English as the primary language spoken at home, lack of family responsibilities or demands, lack of emotional distress, and sense of competency in critical thinking. (Arathuzik & Aber, 1998, p. 119)

CONCLUSIONS

Many similarities exist among diploma, associate, and baccalaureate degree nursing programs regarding predictors of success on the licensure examination. Preadmission criteria such as high school GPA, ACT score, SAT–verbal/math score, and high school rank were found in various combinations to have some correlation with success on the NCLEX–RN. Many of the studies found the NLN test scores in combination with specific nursing theory courses to be the best predictors of NCLEX–RN success. Of particular interest is the finding that clinical nursing course grades were not predictive of passing the NCLEX–RN. This is most probably due to the fact that clinical performance is more difficult to measure objectively, and faculty use various methods of grading performance (i.e., satisfactory/unsatisfactory, pass/fail, numerical and/or letter grades). In contrast, theory courses are more standardized regarding measurement of knowledge and offer more objective information regarding students abilities.

The NLN Baccalaureate Achievement Test and the Mosby Assess Test have been predictive for the majority of programs. It appears that the key to predictive power of these criteria is the model of combination used. Some studies reported the combination of Mosby Assess test and nursing GPA as better predictors than the NLN Achievement Tests and nursing theory courses. Some specific combinations that have been reported in the literature are nursing GPA, nonnursing GPA, and faculty clinical evaluations; nursing course grades, SAT scores, and the NLN Achievement Tests; high school rank, prenursing science grades, and the sophomore GPA; NLN Achievement Tests, nursing GPA, and the Mosby Assess Test. The combination of predictor variables differs from one program to the next, which may be due to factors such as curricular design and characteristics of the student body and/or the faculty.

Numerous studies have been conducted as nursing education programs attempt to identify students at risk for failing the licensure examination and ultimately intervene to help the student prepare for and succeed on the examination. Issues that need to be considered include the organization of the curriculum, program type, background of faculty teaching the major nursing/clinical courses, and composition of the student body. Each program is unique, taking different paths to achieve the same end—successful performance on the NCLEX–RN. This review offers the reader an opportunity to review variables that have had the most success in predicting success on the NCLEX–RN as well as variables that were less likely to predict success. Ultimately, individual programs need to identify which variables most accurately predict success for their own students.

REFERENCES

Aldag, J., & Rose, S. (1983). Relationship of age, American College Testing scores, grade point average and state board examination scores. *Research in Nursing & Health, 6*(2), 69–73.

Alexander, J. E., & Brophy, G. H. (1997). A five year study of graduates' performance on NCLEX–RN. *Journal of Nursing Education, 36*(9), 443–445.

Arathuzik, D., & Aber, C. (1998). Factors associated with National Council Licensure Examination–Registered Nurse success. *Journal of Professional Nursing, 14*(2), 119–126.

Ashley, J. E. (1990). *The effects of three NCLEX preparation programs on nursing knowledge, on test anxiety, and on registered nurse licensure examination performance.* Unpublished doctoral dissertation. Boston College.

Ashley, J. E., & O'Neil, J. (1991). The effectiveness of an intervention to promote successful performance on NCLEX–RN for baccalaureate students at risk for failure. *Journal of Nursing Education, 30*(8), 360–366.

Barkley, T. W., Rhodes, R. S., & Dufour, C. A. (1998). Predictors of success on the NCLEX–RN among baccalaureate nursing students. *Nursing and Health Care Perspectives, 19*(3), 132–136.

Bauwens, E. E., & Gerhard, G. G. (1987). The use of the Watson–Glaser critical thinking appraisal to predict success in a baccalaureate nursing program. *Journal of Nursing Education, 26,* (7), 278–281.

Bell, J. A., & Martindill, C. F. (1976). A cross-validation study for predictors of scores on state board examinations. *Nursing Research, 25*(1), 54–57.

Bersky, A. K., Krawczak, J., & Kumar, T. D. (1998). Computerized clinical simulation testing: A new look for the NCLEX–RN examination? *Nurse Educator, 23*(1), 20–25.

Bosma, J. (1992). The NCLEX–RN in letters to the editor. *Journal of Nursing Education, 31*(7), 291–292.

Boyle, K. K. (1986). Predicting the success of minority students in a baccalaureate nursing program. *Journal of Nursing Education, 25*(5), 186–192.

Breyer, F. J. (1984, April). The comprehensive nursing achievement test as a predictor of performance on the NCLEX–RN. *Nursing & Health Care,* pp. 193–195.

Campbell-Warnock, J., Jones-Dickson, C., & Fields, F. (1993). The NCLEX development process: Some things don't change. *Issues* 5, 6, 8, 9, 10.

Cloud-Hardaway, S. A. (1988). *Relationship among "Mosby's Assess Test" scores, academic performance, and demographic factors and associate degree nursing graduates NCLEX scores.* Unpublished doctoral dissertation, North Texas State University.

Crane, P., Wright, C. R., & Michael, W. B. (1987). School-related variables as predictors of achievement on the national council licensure examination (NCLEX–RN) for a sample of 418 students enrolled in a diploma nursing program. *Educational and Psychological Measurement, 47*(4), 1055–1069.

Deardorff, M., Denner, P., & Miller, C. (1976). Selected National League of Nursing Achievement Test scores as predictors of state board examination scores. *Nursing Research, 25*(1), 35–38.

Dell, M. A., & Halpin, G. (1984). Predictors of success in nursing school and on state board examinations in a predominantly black baccalaureate nursing program. *Journal of Nursing Education, 23*(4), 147–150.

Dell, M. S., & Valine, W. J. (1990). Explaining differences in NCLEX–RN scores with certain cognitive and non-cognitive factors for new baccalaureate nurse graduates. *Journal of Nursing Education, 29*(4), 158–162.

Drake, C. C., & Michael, W. B. (1995). Criterion-related validity of selected achievement measures in the prediction of a passing or failing criterion on the National Council Licensure Examination (NCLEX) for nursing students in a two-year associate degree program. *Educational and Psychological Measurement, 55*(4), 675–679.

Endres, D. (1997). A comparison of predictors of success on NCLEX–RN for African American, foreign-born, and white baccalaureate graduates. *Journal of Nursing Education, 36*(8), 365–371.

Feldt, R. C., & Donahue, J. M. (1989). Predicting nursing GPA and National Council Licensure Examination for Registered Nurses (NCLEX–RN): A thorough analysis. *Psychological Reports, 64*(2), 415–421.

Felts, J. (1986). Performance predictors for nursing courses and NCLEX–RN. *Journal of Nursing Education, 25*, (9), 372–377.

Foti, I., & DeYoung, S. (1991). Predicting success on the National Council Licensure Examination-Registered Nurse: Another piece of the puzzle. *Journal of Professional Nursing, 7*(2), 99–104.

Fowles, E. R. (1992). Predictors of success on NCLEX–RN and within the nursing curriculum: Implications for early intervention. *Journal of Nursing Education, 31*(2), 53–57.

Friedemann, M. L., & Valentine, S. (1988). Success in old and new licensure examinations: Pre-admission factors and academic performance. *Research in Nursing and Health, 11*, 343–350.

Frierson, H., Malone, B., & Shelton, P. (1993). Enhancing NCLEX–RN performance: Assessing a three-pronged intervention approach. *Journal of Nursing Education, 35*(5), 222–224.

Froman, R. D. & Owen, S. V. (1989). Predicting performance on the National Council Licensure Examination. *Western Journal of Nursing Research, 11*(3), 334–346.

Glick, O. J., McClelland, E., & Yang, J. C. (1986). NCLEX–RN: Predicting the performance of graduates of an integrated baccalaureate nursing program. *Journal of Professional Nursing, 2,* 98–103.

Gross, Y. T., Takazawa, E. S., & Rose, C. L. (1987). Critical thinking and nursing education. *Journal of Nursing Education, 26*(8), 317–323.

Halkitus, P. N., & Leahy, J. M. (1993). Computerized adaptive testing: The future is upon us. *Nursing and Health Care, 14*(7), 378–385.

Heupel, C. (1994). A model for intervention and predicting success on the National Council Licensure Examination for Registered Nurses. *Journal of Professional Nursing, 10*(1), 57–60.

Horns, P. N., O'Sullivan, P., & Goodman, R. (1991). The use of progressive indicators as predictors of NCLEX–RN success and performance of BSN graduates. *Journal of Nursing Education, 30*(1), 9–14.

Jenks, J., Selekman, J., Bross, T., & Paquet, M. (1989). Success in NCLEX–RN: Identifying predictors and optimal timing for intervention. *Journal of Nursing Education, 28*(3), 112–118.

Kane, M. T. (1982). The validity of licensure examinations. *American Psychologist, 37*(8), 911–918.

Krupa, K. C., Quick, M. M., & Whitley, T. W. (1988). The effectiveness of nursing grades in predicting performance on the NCLEX–RN. *Journal of Professional Nursing, 4*(4), 294–298.

Lengacher, C. A., & Keller, R. (1990). Academic predictors of success on the NCLEX–RN examination for registered nurses. *Journal of Nursing Education, 29*(4), 163–169.

Marquis, B., & Worth, C. (1992). The relationship among multiple assessments of nursing education outcomes. *Journal of Nursing Education, 31*(1), 33–38.

Matassarin-Jacobs, E. (1989). The nursing licensure process and the NCLEX–RN. *Nurse Educator, 14*(6), 32–35.

McClelland, E., Yang, J. C., & Glick, O. J. (1992). A statewide study of academic variables affecting performance of baccalaureate nursing graduates on licensure examination. *Journal of Professional Nursing, 8*(6), 342–350.

McKinney, J., Small, S., O'Dell, N., & Coonrod, B. A. (1988). Identification of predictors of success for the NCLEX and students at risk for NCLEX failure in a baccalaureate nursing program. *Journal of Professional Nursing, 4,* 55–59.

Melcolm, N., & Bausell, R. B. (1981). The prediction of State Board Test Pool examinations scores within an integrated curriculum. *Journal of Nursing Education, 20*(5), 24–28.

Mills, A. C., Becker, A. M., Sampel, M. E., & Pohlman, V. C.(1992). Success-failure on the National Council Licensure Examination for Registered Nurses by nurse candidates from an accelerated baccalaureate nursing program. *Journal of Professional Nursing, 8*(6), 351–357.

Mills, A. C., Sampel, M. E., Pohlman, V. C., & Becker, A. M. (1992). The odds for success on NCLEX–RN by nurse candidates from a four-year baccalaureate nursing program. *Journal of Nursing Education, 31*(9), 403–408.

National Council of State Boards of Nursing, Inc. (1989). 1990 Marks start of field testing for computerized adaptive testing project. *Issues, 10*(4), 2, 4.

National Council of State Boards of Nursing, Inc. (1990). What affects NCLEX passing rates? *Issues, 11*(4), 10–15.

National Council of State Boards of Nursing, Inc. (1993). Field tests of NCLEX using computerized adaptive testing. *Issues* (special edition), pp. 7, 11, 14.

National Council of State Boards of Nursing, Inc. (1993). A new generation in competence assessment in nursing: Computerized clinical simulation test (CST). *Issues, 14*(1), 1–8.

Outtz, J. H. (1979). Predicting the success on state board examinations for blacks. *Journal of Nursing Education, 18*(9), 35–40.

Payne, M. A., & Duffey, M. A. (1986). An investigation of the predictability of NCLEX scores of BSN graduates using academic predictors. *Journal of Professional Nursing, 2,* 326–332.

Perez, T. L. (1977). Investigation of academic moderator variables to predict success on state board of nursing examinations in a baccalaureate nursing program. *Journal of Nursing Education, 16*(8), 16–23.

Poorman, S. G., & Martin, J. (1991). The role of nonacademic variables in passing the National Council Licensure Examination. *Journal of Professional Nursing, 7*(1), 25–32.

Quick, M. M., Krupa, K. C., & Whitley, T. W. (1985). Using admission data to predict success on the NCLEX-RN in a baccalaureate program. *Journal of Professional Nursing, 1,* 364–368.

Rami, J. S. (1992). Predicting nursing student's success on NCLEX–RN. *ABNF Journal, 3*(3), 67–71.

Schwirian, P. M., Baer, C. L., Basta, S. M., & Larabee, J. G. (1978). Prediction of successful nursing performance (Publication No. 0-245-048). Washington, DC: U.S. Government Printing Office.

Sharp, T. G. (1984). An analysis of the relationship of seven selected variables to State Board Test Pool Examination performance of the University of Tennessee, Knoxville, College of Nursing. *Journal of Nursing Education, 23*(2), 57–63.

Sheil, E. P., & Meisenheimer, C. G. (1992). Helping new graduates succeed at the NCLEX–RN experience, Evaluation of an anxiety-reducing workshop. *Journal of Nursing Staff Development, 8*(5), 213–217.

Stronck, D. R. (1979). Predicting student performance from college admission criteria. *Nursing Outlook, 27*(9), 604–607.

St. Thomas, S. (1982). *An analysis of the relationship between the first semester grade point average and the state board nursing scores of Vermont college graduates.* Unpublished manuscript, Nova University.

Taylor. C. W., Nahm. H., Loy, L., Harms, M., Berthod, J., & Wolfer, J. A. (1966). *Selection and recruitment of nurses and nursing students.* Salt Lake City: University of Utah Press.

Taylor, C. W., Nahm, H., Quinn, M., Harms, M., Mulaik, J., & Mulaik, S. A. (1965). *Report of measurement and predication of nursing performance, Part I.* Salt Lake City: University of Utah.

Veith, S. (1978). Rethinking the integrated curriculum. *Nursing Outlook, 26*(3), 187–190.

Wall, B. M., Miller, D. E. & Widerquist, J. G. (1993). Predictors of success on the newest NCLEX–RN. *Western Journal of Nursing Research, 15*(5), 628–643.

Washburn, G. (1980). Relationship of achievement test scores and state board performance in a diploma nursing program. Doctoral dissertation (No. EDRS-ED203572), Indiana University at South Bend.

Washburn, J., & Short, L. (1992). The NCLEX–RN and nurse educators. *Journal of Nursing Education, 31*(4), 171–174.

Waterhouse, J. K., Carroll, M. C., & Beeman, P. B. (1993). National council licensure examination success: accurate prediction of student performance on the post-1988 examination. *Journal of Professional Nursing, 9*(5), 278–283.

Wells, R. W. (1991). International predictive testing for NCLEX–RN: Rewards and risks. *Nursing and Health Care, 12*(9), 470–473.

Whitley, M., & Chadwick, P. (1986). Baccalaureate education and NCLEX: The causes of success. *Journal of Nursing Education, 25*(3), 94–101.

Woodham, R., & Taube, K. (1986). Relationship of nursing program predictors and success on the NCLEX–RN examination for licensure in a selected associate degree program. *Journal of Nursing Education, 25*(3), 112–117.

Yang, J. C., Glick, O. J., & McClelland, E. (1987). Academic correlates of baccalaureate graduate performance on NCLEX–RN. *Journal of Professional Nursing, 3,* 298–306.

Yocum, C. J. (1987). Statistical approaches to educational program evaluation with new NCLEX score reporting. *Issues 8*(6), 5–7.

Yocum, C. J., & Scherubel, J. C. (1985). Selected pre-admission and academic correlates of success on state board examinations. *Journal of Nursing Education, 24*(6), 244–249.

Younger, J. B., & Grap, M. J. (1992). An epidemiologic study of NCLEX. *Nurse Educator, 17*(2), 24–28.

Zink, M. H. (1991). *Performance of at-risk students of a baccalaureate degree nursing program in selected nursing courses and on the National Council Licensure Examination for Registered Nurses.* Unpublished doctoral dissertation, Ball State University, Indiana.

Chapter 6

Educational Preparation
of Nurse Practitioners
as Advanced-Practice Nurses

COLLEEN KELLER, RN, C, PHD
JUDITH FULLERTON, CNM, PHD, FACNM

INTRODUCTION

Health care trends are increasingly shaping clinical practice, research, and nursing education, particularly in the preparation of clinical practitioners with advanced degrees. In 1991, a major report published by the Pew Health Professions Commission anticipated significant changes in the health care environment, many of which were implemented in the ensuing years. Those changes included the expansion of health care from a focus on the provision of individual care to a system that addresses overall population health; the delivery of curative and preventive services by a judicious provider mix working in ambulatory settings; and systematic measurement of outcomes; quality improvement, standardized practice, and practitioner accountability (The Pew Health Professions Commission, 1991). These changes, coupled with the information and biotechnological explosion and consumer empowerment, have created the need for nurses with advanced-practice skills far beyond diagnostic and technical expertise (Safriet, 1992). Expert educators believe that practitioners prepared for practice in this environment should study advanced nursing, research, health promotion and maintenance, data acquisition, counseling and advice, appropriate referral, economics of care, and multi/interdisciplinary practice (Booth, 1995; Rasch & Frauman, 1996).

Periodically, any discipline must analyze critically the education of those in the profession for relevancy and accountability in content, and appropriateness of the context of the education within a changing sociocultural milieu. This paper examines the research focused on the educational preparation and role delineation of nurse practitioners (NPs) as advanced-practice nurses (APNs) (a relatively recent and overarching term that encompasses the various clinical nurse specialist [CNS], NP, and certified nurse midwifery [CNM] titles) (American Association of Colleges of Nursing [AACN], 1996; Rasch & Frauman, 1996). Existing meta-analytical reviews indicate that the advanced-practice nursing literature prior to 1980 focused primarily on the emerging or expanding role of the NP, CNM, and nurse anesthetist and on the comparison of patient outcomes of NPs and CNMs relative to physicians. Research-based literature concerning education and clinical practice is more recent; thus, only the literature from 1980 through the present was reviewed. Two articles prior to 1980 are included in the bibliography and are noted for the seminal work they represent in evaluating the care provided by NPs compared to physicians.

METHOD

Many investigations of topics of clinical and scientific interest are being synthesized for rapid and sensible utilization. Meta-analysis is the most recognized approach to integrating studies; however, study designs in some content areas do not lend themselves to statistical meta-analysis. A variation of the meta-analytical approach has been developed to allow a rigorous examination of reports in these areas. This approach, called nonstatistical meta-analysis, was developed by Bland, Meurer, and Maldonado (1995) and adapted for the current report. This technique is presented fully elsewhere, but briefly it includes literature retrieval, literature coding, rating for quality, annotation of high-quality references, and synthesis of the basic results of each study.

Retrieval of the Literature

A computerized on-line search of nursing, medicine, and allied health literature was conducted; the databases used included ERIC, Medline, and the Cumulative Index of Nursing and Allied Health Literature (CINAHL). The topical heading of "nurse practitioner" was modified by keywords designed to include studies that focused on education, educational methods, standards of practice, NP utilization, and statistics (including "manpower") and policy trends. A similar search was conducted under the heading of "midwifery" in order to capture nurse-midwifery literature that may have been published in journals of the allied health professions. The abstract of each article identified in this search was reviewed for relevance and retrieval. 189 articles were identified.

The majority of articles retrieved were editorial or anecdotal concerning practice roles, clinical experiences, and issues related to the educational preparation of the NP, CNS, and CNM. To be selected for inclusion in this review, the article had to include information about the research design and the statistical approach used to gather and analyze data.

Literature Coding

Each article was sorted for inclusion within one of three primary topical domains. The first domain focused on the historical development of NP education and the evolution and evaluation of the role (AACN, 1996; Abdellah, 1982; Fenton & Brykczynski, 1993; Rolfe & Phillips, 1997; Shah, Bruttomesso, Sullivan, & Lanttanzio, 1997). Studies within this domain focused on the efficacy of the APN in clinical practice (Courtney & Rice, 1997) and the impact of the NP on health care costs (Office of Technology Assessment, 1986; Sackett, Spitzer, Gent & Roberts, 1974; Spitzer et al., 1974). Some of these effectiveness studies also included a comparison to physician or physician assistant providers (McCaig, Hooker, Sekscenski, & Woodwell, 1998). This body of research provides important reference data and has itself been subject to recent meta-analytical review (Brown & Grimes, 1995).

The second domain addressed investigations concerning the content of curricula of APN education programs. Research in this domain included the investigation of teaching methods, the process of clinical teaching, and evaluation strategies.

The third domain included investigations on the role delineation of advanced, nursing practice. These studies provided important information concerning revisions in curricula that accompanied the expansion of NP practice, including the expansion of clinical practice into both remote and underserved geographic environments, such as rural health and community-focused primary care. Other studies focused on the current controversy over the merging of the educational preparation and practice roles of the NP and the CNS (Lindeke, Canedy & Kay, 1997; Rasch & Frauman, 1996; Thibodeau & Hawkins, 1994).

Rating for Quality

Each article within the three target domains was then reviewed with regard to the rigor of the scientific design (for experimental studies) and/or the comprehensiveness of the report. Methodological considerations included sample size, quality of the design elements, strength of instrumentation, and statistical analysis and outcome variables. Those articles that were primarily descriptive narratives were given lower priority for inclusion than were articles that analyzed the issues under discussion. These decisions were made independently by the two authors. The ultimate criterion was not to be all-inclusive but, instead, to be selective and representative of the scope of the literature, and the depth of the most instructive research studies. 31 articles were considered acceptable in terms of the criteria.

Annotation of References

Annotation of articles selected for review was conducted with each author working separately. Posthoc discussion between the authors was oriented toward achieving a measure of interrater reliability for the annotated data. 21 studies are annotated under the domain of NP curriculum and role delineation/scope of practice. Articles in the first domain are not presented in table format because a majority of this information is available in the recent report by Brown and Grimes (1995).

Synthesis of the Basic Results of Each Study

The results of the research concerning the education of advanced practice nurses appear in Tables 6–1 and 6–2.

RESULTS

Historical Development of Nurse Practitioner Education

The need to increase the availability and accessibility of skilled health care providers has guided the curricula of NP education since its inception in Colorado in 1965 (Ford & Silver, 1967). Nurse midwifery education and nurse anesthesia education in the United States have a longer history; however, the advent of NP education helped to raise the consciousness of the health care system about the contributions of these advanced-practice nurse specialties. By the 1970s, more than 500 programs prepared nurses as advanced practitioners (Garland & Marchione, 1982). Papers concerning the early phases of advanced-practice education were primarily focused on the content of programs as being designed to meet the needs of underserved individuals and communities

TABLE 6–1.
Summary of Research in the Education of Advanced-Practice Nurses: Curriculum

Author/Date	Sample	Purpose	Method	Results
Brereton (1995)	4 nurse teachers, 76 students, 17 mentors from a single college in England.	Examine the relationship between the theory of communication/interpersonal skills and practice of those skills, and identify the factors that influenced the relationship between theory and practice.	Qualitative survey using content analysis.	Although difficult to measure, the theory underpinning communication and interpersonal skills was valued and applied to practice. There was a potential theory practice gap related to mentor's knowledge of curriculum and the communication theories used in the curriculum.
Bramble (1994)	18 NP students (controls), 11 NP students (experimental subjects).	An objective structural clinical assessment (OSCA) was examined to determine the effect that participation in this clinical simulation would have on cognitive and clinical competency.	Quasi-experimental: experimental = OSCA, control = lecture/discussion method.	OSCA simulation did not lead to significantly better cognitive or clinical performance than the lecture discussion method.
Busen & Jones (1995)	21 PNP graduate students.	Examine personal variables with respect to leadership potential.	Descriptive survey.	Personality type was not related to ability to function as change agent. There was no difference in a graduate's ability to deal with conflict reduction or function as a change agent prior to and after completion of a program.
Davis et al. (1993)	15 NP preceptors (11 NP, 4 MW).	Explore strategies expert preceptors used in working with graduate students within the clinical setting.	Qualitative/content analysis.	Identified preceptor styles (incremental structure or "sink or swim"). Identified four patterns of teaching strategies: role modeling, charting, pre–post conferences, and guided questioning.
Forbes et al. (1990)	108 schools with graduate NP and CNS programs (317 programs).	Compare core curriculum of NP to CNS core curriculum.	Survey.	NP programs emphasize pharmacology, primary care, physical assessment, health promotion, nutrition, and history taking. Other core curricula were similar.

TABLE 6–1.
Summary of Research in the Education of Advanced-Practice Nurses: Curriculum (Continued)

Author/Date	Sample	Purpose	Method	Results
Fullerton et al. (1993)	17 nurse midwife students, 8 nurse midwife faculty.	Assess the reliability of a single component of a performance evaluation protocol ("faculty impression score").	Evaluation protocol.	Test–retest reliability was .90 to .97; student feedback was provided in the conceptual framework of the evaluation process; evaluation protocol was behaviorally anchored and criterion referenced.
Jones (1992)	97 PNPs who were members at the New York Chapter of NAPNAP (64 respondents).	Examine education and training in injury prevention and control as used in clinical practice.	Survey.	NPs received injury prevention in NP education; the majority used this education in practice.
Lange et al. (1997)	9 NP students from one western state NP program.	Determine the effect of a computer-mediated training program on NP students' diagnostic inquiry skills.	2×2 random design; students as their own controls.	The computer-mediated program increased diagnostic decision-making capability somewhat; prior experience in providing general nursing care to patients with that same diagnosis increased effects of Iliad training.
Morgan & Trolinger (1994)	112 directors of ambulatory care NP programs.	Determine the amount and characteristics of clinical education.	Survey, 53% response rate.	Subjects had an average of 597 clinical hours (range: 192–1,600 hours), clinical training in conjunction with medical PA students, and clinical experience mixed among hospital outpatient clinics, public community clinics, and for-profit/nonprofit clinics.
Murdock & Neafsey (1995)	36 APNs enrolled in pharmacology CE course.	Assess the usefulness of measurements.	Pre- and posttest design.	Participants incurred knowledge and self-sufficiency in evaluating practice outcome following CE pharmacology course. Confidence to prescribe is determined by change between pre- and posttest scores.
Swingler (1994)	102 midwife recipients of the Neonopoly game (79 respondents).	Test a board game (Neonopoly) that helps midwives learn the principles of neonatal primary care.	Survey.	Game aided learning, stimulated discussion.

TABLE 6–1.
Summary of Research in the Education of Advanced-Practice Nurses: Curriculum (Continued)

Author/Date	Sample	Purpose	Method	Results
Talashek et al. (1995)	16 FNP students, 8 NPs.	Evaluate competencies in substance abuse and dependency, and test student clinical performance scale.	Pre- and posttesting on multiple-choice exam clinical performance evaluation.	FNP students who received special education on substance abuse were somewhat knowledgeable (on exam) and more likely to conduct patient assessments (in practice) than prescribing ANPs.
Walsh & Jaspan (1990)	13 lay midwives who were also CNMs; 63 NMW educators.	Identify perceived learning needs of students with midwifery experience who enter nurse midwifery education programs.	Descriptive survey.	Nurse midwifery educators follow a more culturally and socially acceptable route to professional preparation.

APN = advanced-practice nurse
CE = continuing education
CNM = certified nurse midwife
CNS = clinical nurse specialist
FNP = family nurse practitioner
MW = midwife

NAPNAP = National Association of Pediatric Nurse Associates and Practitioners
NMW = nurse midwife
NP = nurse practitioner
PA = physician's assistant
PNP = pediatric nurse practitioner

TABLE 6–2.
Summary of Research in the Education of Advanced-Practice Nurses: Role Delineation and the Scope of Practice

Author/Date	Sample	Purpose	Method	Results
Batey & Holland (1983)	5 states—legal authority for prescriptive practice as cited in state regulations.	Determine how the degree of rigidity or flexibility within the practice act affects actual NP prescribing practice.	"Natural experiment" observation.	In states that grant NPs more authority within the practice act, more prescribing practice occurs. Clinical preceptorship in underserved areas; clinical preceptorship in areas where students lived.
Flowers et al. (1989)	1000 ob/gyn NPs.	Investigate ways in which ob/gyn nurses who are in current practice acquire new knowledge as a basis for practice change.	Survey.	Continuing education conferences and discussion with colleagues were two most important strategies.
Fowkes et al. (1994)	51 ANP programs (170 interviews with faculty, students graduates, employers).	Determine the strategies used to prepare ANPs for medically underserved areas.	Interview response rate.	Programs with a mission statement to train ANPs for underserved populations/areas used strategies to accomplish that mission.
Hafferty & Goldberg (1986)	231 graduates of primary care associate program.	Examine factors related to retention of providers in the catchment area where they had resided before attending school.	Descriptive survey.	Matching students with preceptors for clinical experience in location of residence assisted retention.
Hupcey (1994)	13 nursing schools, 94 ANP students.	Describe master's-level NP student's expectations of the role behavior of a NP, and identify factors within the socialization process that seem to influence these expectations.	Survey (questionnaire): socialization process, role expectations.	Opportunity to practice selected role behaviors in clinical setting influenced student expectation of role behaviors. NP as teacher ranked as highest valued role behavior. Role expectation included evaluating patient care and formulating problem list. Technical aspects of role behaviors were highly valued.

TABLE 6–2.
Summary of Research in the Education of Advanced-Practice Nurses: Role Delineation and the Scope of Practice (Continued)

Author/Date	Sample	Purpose	Method	Results
Hupcey (1990)	80 NPs in Pennsylvania (all specialties).	Compare the role of master's-prepared and non-master's-prepared practitioners, and to compare actual and ideal role behaviors between the two groups.	Survey (questionnaire): demographics, role performance.	No difference in actual role behaviors as a function of academic degree level. Master's-prepared NPs rated technical skills to be of higher importance than non-master's-prepared NPs.
Lindeke et al. (1997)	15 NPs originally prepared in the CNS role.	Identify similarities and differences between NP and CNS roles as perceived by individuals who had preparation in both APN specialties.	Interviews.	Differences in the two specialties were most distinct in the NONPF domains of management of client health–illness studies and professional role.
Wilbur et al. (1990)	113 FNPs who had graduated 1–11 years earlier from a single graduate program.	Follow-up of FNP graduates to determine retention in primary care practice settings.	Survey.	For both first and present jobs, the majority were providing direct patient care as a primary care provider or practicing in an indirect role.

APN = advanced-practice nurse
CNS = clinical nurse specialist
FNP = family nurse practitioner
NONPF = National Organization of Nurse Practitioner Faculties
NP = nurse practitioner

(Koch, Pazaki, & Campbell, 1992). As analyzed by Koch and colleagues (1992), education articles described advanced-practice nursing programs that emphasized primary health care and leadership issues concerning joint practice and hierarchical relationships with physician providers. Two large investigations concerning the early education and role development of advanced-practice nursing are noteworthy: the Burlington randomized clinical trial of NPs and the policy analysis conducted by the Office of Technology Assessment (Office of Technology Assessment, 1986; Sackett et al., 1974; Spitzer et al., 1974). These reports present similar conclusions: that NPs and nurse midwives provide equivalently competent clinical care, particularly in well and chronically ill populations, when compared to their physician counterparts. These seminal studies have been duplicated exhaustively in the ensuing 20 years, with varied samples of patient settings, outcomes, and designs.

Research concerning the historical development of the advanced-practice nurse has focused on the efficacy of care provided in terms of cost and patient outcomes. While results are not explicit, one can infer that educational programs emphasized clinical skill acquisition in health and illness assessment and patient management of health problems. Role delineation in a labor market and professional competitive environment contributed to anecdotal literature emphasizing educational models that included leadership and interdisciplinary practice (Koch et al., 1992).

In 1995, Brown and Grimes conducted a meta-analysis of the research in comparing patient outcomes between NPs, midwives, and physicians. Their analysis offers a succinct summary of the historical literature. These authors concluded that the majority of studies were not generalizable because they lacked randomization of patients to providers, used approaches to compute the cost of care that limited interpretations about the cost-effectiveness of advanced nurse practitioners, or listed outcome measures that could not precisely determine the equivalency of patient outcomes between providers. The authors did acknowledge that advanced-practice nurses provide care that is equivalent to or better than physician care in situations in which the nurses were prepared, such as health promotion and care of minor acute and stable chronic conditions (Brown & Grimes, 1995).

The Content of Advanced-Nurse Practitioner Education

The studies that addressed the curriculum of nurse practitioners had no clear focus or theme. The research appearing in the literature was primarily descriptive using convenience samples. Only four studies indicated an experimental or quasi-experimental design for comparing two educational strategies for specific content acquisition. The literature related to educational preparation had three areas of focus: general curriculum content (Brereton, 1995; Busen & Jones, 1995; Forbes, Rafson, Spross, & Kozlowski, 1990; Walsh & Jaspan, 1990), specific curriculum content (Jones, 1992; Murdock & Neafsey, 1995; Swingler, 1994; Talashek, Gerace, Miller, & Lindsey, 1995), and clinical education

(Bramble, 1994; Davis, Sawin, & Dunn, 1993; Fullerton, Piper, & Hunter, 1993; Lange et al., 1997; Morgan & Trolinger, 1994).

Curriculum Content. The National League for Nursing (NLN) standards for clinical education of adult nurse practitioners do not provide specific guidelines for the duration of education programs. However, some professional organizations and some state licensing agencies have addressed this issue (Shah, Sullivan, Lattanzio, & Bruttomesso, 1993). For example, the National Association of Pediatric Nurse Associates and Practitioners (NAPNAP) (1996) and the National Organization of Nurse Practitioner Faculties (NONPF) (1995) have cited a minimum of 500 hours, noting that some specialties may require more than this. Morgan and Trolinger (1994), from a survey of 112 NP programs, examined the length of clinical education of primary care nurse practitioner students. This survey revealed that the issue of graduate education versus certificate education did not determine the length of clinical training; certificate programs exceeded graduate programs in length of clinical training.

The American Nurses Association's Council of Clinical Nurse Specialists and Council of Primary Health Care NPs conducted a survey of all graduate programs in the United States offering CNS and/or NP preparation. One hundred eight schools offering 317 programs responded to the survey. It was found that the core curriculum of NP graduate programs places more emphasis on pharmacology, primary care, physical assessment, health promotion, nutrition, and history taking as compared to curricula of CNS programs. All other required core courses were similar between the two advanced practice curricula (Forbes et al., 1990).

A survey of clinical practice concerning childhood injury prevention and the education underpinning that content was conducted by Jones (1992). Sixty-four pediatric nurse practitioners (PNPs) belonging to the greater New York chapter of their professional association were surveyed. All of those surveyed received preparation in injury prevention, and all used this knowledge to provide parent/patient teaching of child restraints, smoke detectors, safe water temperature, and firearms.

Specific content in the area of substance abuse was provided to 16 family nurse practitioner (FNP) students. These students were found to be somewhat more knowledgeable in the content area as measured by pre-and posttesting, and were significantly more likely to use this knowledge in clinical practice as assessed on a structured clinical performance examination when compared to eight practicing FNPs (Talashek et al., 1995).

Recently, the revised *Curriculum Guidelines and Program Standards for Nurse Practitioner Education* were published by the NONPF (1995). The educational model proposed for curricula is based on research on the clinical practice of experienced nurses (Benner, 1984; Brykczynski, 1989). This model includes "domains," which are clusters of competencies that have similar functions, and "competencies," an interpretively defined area of skilled knowledge (NONPF, 1995). Six domains of practice are identified in this model, with subsequent delineation of competencies to guide curricula. They are management of client health/illness status, the nurse–client relationship, the teaching–coaching function, professional role, managing and negotiating health care delivery systems, and monitoring and ensuring the quality of health care practice. Among the competencies for each domain are the applications of the theoretical and scientific underpinnings of advanced nursing practice. While this model and an earlier version of it (NONPF, 1995) have been available to advanced-practice nurse educators, the extant literature concerning research in this specialized area of nursing education has largely ignored the suggested competencies and their theoretical foundations. Research concerning the application of these competencies is absent in educational research on NPs.

Clinical Teaching and Evaluation. NP skills and decision-making abilities are acquired in the clinical arena, primarily under the tutelage of an expert practitioner in primary care or midwifery. Preceptors provide an important part of the education of advanced-practice nurses. Other than anecdotal information concerning the desirable qualities of preceptors, very little research has been conducted in this area. Davis et al. (1993) examined teaching strategies used by expert NPs. Qualitative methods using content analysis guided 15 interviews of expert NP preceptors examining teaching strategies. Overall teaching strategies were the manipulation of the clinical environment and optimization of interventions among the client, student, and preceptor. Two preceptor styles were identified: one providing incremental structure to the student, and the other following the "sink or swim" approach. The investigators identified three patterns of orientation strategies: general orientation, identification of students' strengths, and orientation to preceptor style. This investigation underscored the importance of matching students' learning styles with preceptors' teaching styles.

The relationship between theory and practice in communication and interpersonal relationships was examined by Brereton (1995). Using qualitative methods with content analysis, Brereton interviewed four nurse midwife faculty, 76 students, and 17 mentors in the United Kingdom concerning the use of theoretical underpinnings in practice. While all study participants acknowledged the value of theory to practice, theory was considered "idealistic." Faculty found it difficult to assess whether students were using theory-based practice, and they relied on mentors to assess the use of theory.

Busen and Jones (1995) hypothesized that personal characteristics, such as personality type, self-esteem, and learning style, were related to the leadership potential of 21 PNP graduates. Several instruments were thought to characterize personal characteristics and leadership potential: the Learning Style Inventory, the Meyers–Briggs Personality Inventory, Hoffmeister's Self-Esteem Questionnaire, the Conflict Mode Instrument, and Hall and Williams's Change Agent Questionnaire. All of these instruments were administered prior to and following the PNP program. The PNP students in the sample used personal warmth rather than objective analysis in problem solving and human interactions and preferred concrete learning situations rather than abstract ones. There was no difference in the graduates' ability to resolve conflict or function as a change agent following the program. The authors did not delineate what curricular or clinical experiences would contribute, either theoretically or empirically, to changes in leadership potential.

The potential conflict between lay midwives entering nurse midwife education programs and the nurse midwife faculty led to the examination of attitudes and learning needs of the lay midwives (Walsh & Jaspan, 1990). The faculty responding to the survey ($N = 63$) reported that the lay midwife students needed scientific methods and relied on experience rather than data collection in decision making. Lay midwife students ($N = 13$) reported they needed information in areas not addressed in lay midwifery, such as pharmacology and high-risk care.

A board game was developed to provide clinical simulation and decision making in neonatal primary care (Swingler, 1994). The game, called Neonopoly, involves players moving around a board that simulates a neonatal primary care environment. Problem-oriented clinical questions guide the participants in health prevention/promotion aspects of neonatology. 79 questionnaires were administered to midwives learning neonatal primary care through use of Neonopoly. Users reported that the game aided learning and stimulated discussion and interest in neonatal primary care.

A computerized diagnostic reasoning expert system ("Iliad") was used to teach NP students to reach a disease-focused diagnostic decision (Lange et al., 1997). This computer program presents clinical studies in the form of history and physical examination data and diagnostic test findings. Students must draw inferences about the relationship between these data and a probable diagnosis. Nine NP students each completed four case management studies using the Iliad method and four in a conventional study mode. Use of the Iliad system did improve NP students' diagnostic reasoning skills somewhat. These training effects were enhanced if the NP students had encountered similar patient problems during their experience in nursing.

Because the evaluation of student performance may not be reliable and valid during a faculty site visit, and because of the variety of clinical situations, NP students may not always receive adequate formative feedback on clinical practice (Bramble, 1994). The Objective Structured Clinical Assessment (OSCA) is a method of assessing clinical performance that is objective rather than subjective. The method emphasizes the student's ability to obtain a focused patient history or perform a limited physical exam, which is evaluated against preformed criteria. An examination of OSCA was conducted using a quasi-experimental design (18 experimental subjects, 11 controls). Dependent measures were scores on midterm exams and clinical competency as rated by preceptor evaluation. Participation in an OSCA did not contribute to significantly better cognitive or clinical performance.

Murdock and Neafsey (1995) studied the use of self-efficacy in evaluating a continuing education pharmacology course for advanced-practice nurses.

Self-efficacy was defined as the confidence in one's ability to prescribe and included knowledge of drug action and side effects, adverse drug reactions, and ability to monitor drug therapy. Thirty-six APNs completed pretest–posttest measures; 20 completed two-year follow-ups. Both knowledge and self-efficacy scores improved following the course, but there were low correlations between knowledge and self-efficacy scores, suggesting that the measures may tap different dimensions of learning outcomes.

Clinical evaluation of practitioner students and, in particular, the need for interrater reliability between faculty in the evaluation process stimulated the development and testing of a clinical performance tool for nurse midwifery students (Fullerton et al., 1993). This investigation examined the interfaculty reliability of a "faculty impression score" on 10 personal and professional performance domains. The content validity of the tool was based on a review of nurse midwifery literature, such as standards of nurse midwifery practice. Two reliability trials yielded reliability coefficients of .90 and .97.

In summary, the literature concerning advanced nurse practice curricula and the process of clinical teaching and evaluation has primarily focused on developing and describing new methods and measures and reviewing the utility of these strategies. There has been little focus on development, testing, or dissemination of a particular or unique theory-based model for NP education. The recent work by the NONPF professional organization is a singular and important exception. Recent policy debate about requiring the master's degree for entry into advanced-nurse practice is not well informed by extant research. Current literature does not address the unique and critical elements that the curriculum of the graduate degree program contributes to the safety and efficacy of NP practice.

Role Delineation and Role Expansion

Studies cited in this category included articles that primarily addressed the range of activities which NPs included in their scope of practice and the expansion of curriculum content relevant to the geographic and/or demographic profiles of the communities in which they chose to practice. The education of NPs is a response to the need to increase the availability and accessibility of skilled primary care providers. Thus, some research on scope of research includes that of practice site choices. All studies reviewed in this category were descriptive and used convenience samples.

There were a few attempts to correlate educational preparation with practice skills and practice sites. The process of role socialization by NP students and the influence of socialization on their role expectations was examined among NP students enrolled in a graduate program (Hupcey, 1994). 13 schools and 94 students participated in the survey. An instrument that measured the socialization process and role expectations was administered to final-semester students. The results indicated that NP students placed great importance on the technical aspects of the role behaviors, such as evaluating care and developing a problem list. Only one socialization factor influenced role expectation: the opportunity to practice selected role behaviors in the clinical setting.

A second study by the same author (Hupcey, 1990) investigated actual and ideal role behaviors as perceived by master's-prepared and non-master's-prepared NPs. Results of a survey of 80 NPs indicated that master's-prepared NPs valued technical behaviors even more highly than did non-master's-prepared practitioners. Survey participants placed less value on skills in research and theory.

Preparing practitioners to work in medically underserved areas has been the focus of some studies. Fowkes, Gamel, Wilson, and Garcia (1994) examined the effectiveness of recruitment, educational, and deployment strategies that programs used to prepare NPs for medically underserved areas. Fifty-one programs were surveyed: one third of these had a rural focus. Three programs had 80% ethnic minority students, while 16 programs had 14% ethnic minority students. Programs with mission statements directed toward training APNs for underserved populations guided strategic efforts to recruit and deploy graduates to these areas. Thirty-one percent of the programs located in target areas increased the potential for retaining graduates to live in those areas; 41% required a 1- to 3-month preceptorship at underserved sites. Most programs included cultural themes in their curriculum. Programs that were most successful in preparing students to work in underserved sites were those with a clear and direct mission to do so.

Hafferty and Goldberg (1986) also examined strategies for the retention of nonphysician health care providers. They examined the characteristics of physician assistant and NP providers that contributed to the graduates' establishment of a practice within the catchment areas where they resided prior to entering school. This survey of 210 students attending the Primary Care Associate Program at Stanford University Medical Center indicated that students who obtained preclinical training away from home exhibited a high degree of retention to their original catchment area and a high rate of return to the catchment area for preceptorship experience.

Wilbur, Zoeller, Talashek, and Sullivan (1990) surveyed 113 FNPs who had graduated from one to 11 years previously from a single graduate program. The study demonstrated a high rate of retention in direct or indirect clinical practice and a very high rate of retention within communities contiguous to the educational program area.

Batey and Holland (1983) reported one of the earliest evaluations of the impact of state-by-state regulatory differences in prescriptive authority on actual NP practice patterns. Findings of this early study indicated a direct correlation between respect for the capabilities of the NP, which was an emerging role at the time of the study, and liberal prescriptive authority. The study did not address issues of quality in prescribing practice.

Flowers, Gay, Buckner, and Lavender (1989) conducted a national study of 1,000 ob/gyn NPs to determine how ob/gyn NPs made practice change. The survey research indicated that attendance at continuing education conferences and discussions with colleagues were the most important sources of information that NPs incorporated into their patient-management strategies.

Some of the more scientific examinations concerned the role delineation and distinction between CNSs and NPs. Two qualitative studies that used the same methodology and conceptual framework were compared, using the situation as the unit of analysis (Fenton & Bryczynski, 1993). Along with the seven domains identified by Benner (1984), these authors identified two more. The management of health/illness status was identified for the NP subjects, and the consulting role was identified by the CNS subjects. The authors concluded that the CNS role attempts to distinguish between medicine and nursing and keep the roles distinct, while the NP role attempts to blend aspects of medicine and nursing through a nursing perspective (Fenton & Bryczynski, 1993).

Lindeke and colleagues (1997) interviewed 15 NPs whose initial advanced-practice preparation was in the clinical nurse specialist role. The NPs shared the perception that transition to the NP role involved increased role autonomy and clinical decision-making responsibilities. The authors urged that CNS and NP role components be made explicit within advanced-practice graduate nursing curriculum content in order to retain the uniqueness, specificity, and depth of knowledge that presently delineates the two specialty practices.

In summary, the earliest literature on the emerging role of the NP focused on the expansion of that role, and most recent literature has focused on affirming and confirming the role of the advanced-practice nurse in the rapidly changing health care system. The majority of these studies do not distinguish among NPs by title or educational level of role preparation: therefore, these studies will not fully inform contemporary health policy debate concerning the NP role and function.

CONCLUSIONS

This review was intended to synthesize the body of research that underpins NP education. Research studies selected for this review were those that focused on educational evaluation models, documentation of the structure and process of curriculum change, and selected outcome measures such as quality of care and retention in practice. The review presented early literature about the historical development of the NP role but did not emphasize the emerging role-change proposals, as that body of literature is also primarily anecdotal.

An exhaustive search of the NP education literature yielded one theory-based research study (Brereton, 1995). The vast majority of reports over the past 16 years were descriptive or comparative and addressed selected topics within a specialty curriculum (Bramble, 1994; Forbes et al., 1990; Jones, 1992; Morgan & Trolinger, 1994; Murdock & Neafsey, 1995). There are a few evaluation studies, but most of them are short-term assessments of the effectiveness of a new educational strategy or a new way to measure clinical performance (Davis et al., 1993; Fullerton et al., 1993; Lange et al., 1997; Swingler, 1994; Walsh & Jaspan, 1990). A few articles presented reports of new educational models; however, these reports were descriptive and not evaluative.

A few studies focused on the issues of NP deployment to underserved areas (Fowkes et al., 1994; Hafferty & Goldberg, 1996). These studies, however, did not explore all the complex variables contributing to choice of practice sites. None of the studies focused on the merging of NP and CNS roles addressed this particular issue.

The literature search showed that the majority of research studies are focused on the satisfaction with care given by NPs as compared to physician providers, the cost benefit of NP care as compared to other health care providers, health management by NPs compared to providers in several allied health fields, and prescriptive practices (Brown & Grimes, 1995; Sackett et al., 1974; Spitzer et al., 1974). These utilitarian studies are, of course, very important; nevertheless, these studies would be strengthened by a corollary body of research that documents the fundamental soundness of contemporary and emerging approaches to NP education.

RECOMMENDATIONS FOR RESEARCH

This review of research in nursing education concerning the NP role and function offers a clear direction for further inquiry. Because sufficient numbers of APNs are now making a contribution in diverse geographic settings and among ethnically and culturally diverse clientele, large-sample and randomized designs are feasible and should be strongly encouraged. Studies conducted among smaller samples should clearly focus on the several elements that are of critical importance to aggregate (meta-analytical) review: a clear delineation of the practice activities that are assessed as outcome measures, and definitive measures of the cost, not charges, of care. Some clear measure of the process of care should also be included in these studies. Current research does not clarify the essence of the difference among APNs and physicians in the process of care, a difference that has long been postulated.

Further research focused on the content and process of NP education must be directed toward identification, development, or confirmation of theory-based models for curriculum design and evaluation strategies. The NONPF guidelines (1995) were the first example of inductively generated recommendations for curriculum content and process. These guidelines, based on the seminal work of Benner (1984), will also need to be tested as the APN role continues to evolve in the contemporary health care system.

Clinical teaching and evaluation can be improved through research that identifies and confirms the methods and strategies through which students are best prepared to assume the NP role. A few studies were found in this review that focused on the ways by which practitioners gain requisite knowledge and abilities or are fostered in the development of critical thinking skills. Only one study (Brereton, 1995) examined the use of theory in nurse practitioner education.

A salient omission in the studies reviewed was the use of research in NP education: both the utilization of research as the empirical basis of practice and the acquisition of research skills. There was no evidence in the entire retrieval of literature that there was a "science" underpinning NP practice. Rather, there was mention of the acquisition of technical skills and role behaviors (Bramble, 1994; Brereton, 1995; Murdock & Neafsey, 1995; Swingler, 1994; Talashek et al., 1995).

Future studies of the role of the advanced-practice nurse will need to be premised upon a clear definition of the NP title, by education and scope of practice. This review identified two qualitative studies that offered some clear distinction between, and recommended future direction for, the role of the CNS and the NP (Fenton & Brykczynski, 1993; Lindeke et al., 1997). This role distinction is likely a critical factor, given emerging trends. If both categories of APNs are important, then future research must provide clear documentation of process and outcome data to support the distinctive contribution of the role. This documentation will necessarily also include cost-effectiveness analyses and assessment of the quality of care.

REFERENCES

Abdellah, F. G. (1982). The nurse practitioner 17 years later: Present and emerging issues. *Inquiry, 19,* 105–116.

American Association of Colleges of Nursing. (1996). Position statement: Certification and regulation of advanced practice nurses. *Journal of Professional Nursing, 12*(3), 184–186.

The Association of Faculties of Pediatric Nurse Associate/Practitioner Programs and the National Association of Pediatric Nurse Associatesa and Practitioners. (1996). *Standards of practice for PNP/As.* Cherry Hill, NJ.

Batey, M. V., & Holland, J. M. (1983). The impact of structured autonomy accorded through state regulatory policies on nurses prescribing practices. *Image, 15*(3), 84–89.

Benner, P. E. (1984). *From novice to expert: Excellence and power in clinical nursing practice.* Menlo Park, CA: Addison-Wesley.

Bland, C. J., Meurer, L. N., & Maldonado, G. (1995). A systematic approach to conducting a non-statistical meta-analysis of research literature. *Academic Medicine, 70*(7), 642–653.

Booth, R. Z. (1995). Leadership challenges for NP faculty. *Nurse Practitioner, 20*(4), 52–58.

Bramble, K. (1994). Nurse practitioner education: Enhancing performance through the use of objective structured clinical assessment. *The Journal of Nursing Education, 33*(2), 59–65.

Brereton, M. L. (1995). Communication in nursing: The theory–practice relationship. *Journal of Advanced Nursing, 21,* 314–324.

Brown, S. A., & Grimes, D. E. (1995). A meta-analysis of NPs and nurse midwives in primary care. *Nursing Research, 64*(6), 332–339.

Brykczynski, K. A. (1989). An interpretive study describing the clinical judgment of NPs. *Scholarly Inquiry for Nursing Practice: An International Journal, 3*(2), 113–120.

Busen, N. H., & Jones, M. E. (1995). Leadership development: Educating NPs for the future. *Journal of the American Academy of Nurse Practitioners, 7*(3), 111–117.

Courtney, R., & Rice, C. (1997). Investigation of nurse-practitioner patient interactions: Using the nurse practitioner rating form. *The Nurse Practitioner, 22*, 2, 46–65.

Davis, M. S., Sawin, K. J., & Dunn, M. (1993). Teaching strategies used by expert NPs: A qualitative study. *Journal of the American Academy of Nurse Practitioners, 5*(1), 27–33.

Fenton, M. V., & Brykczynski, K. A. (1993). Qualitative distinctions and similarities in the practice of clinical nurse specialists and nurse practitioners. *Journal of Professional Nursing, 61*, 313–326.

Flowers, J. S., Gay, J. T., Buckner E. B., & Lavender, M. G. (1989). How obstetric/gynecologic nurse practitioners make practice changes: A national study. *Journal of the American Academy of Nurse Practitioners, 1*(4), 132–136.

Forbes, K. E., Rafson, J., Spross, J. A., & Kozlowski, D. (1990). Clinical nurse specialist and nurse practitioner core curricula survey results. *Nurse Practitioner, 15*(4), 43–48.

Ford, L., & Silver, H. (1967). The pediatric nurse practitioner in Colorado. *American Journal of Nursing, 67*, 1443–1444.

Fowkes, V. K., Gamel, N. N., Wilson, S. R., & Garcia, R. D. (1994). Effectiveness of educational strategies preparing physician assistants, NPs, and certified nurse midwives for underserved areas. *Public Health Reports, 109*(5), 673–682.

Fullerton, J. T., Piper, D. M., & Hunter, L. (1993). Development of a single component of a performance evaluation protocol. The Faculty Impression Score. *Journal of Nurse Midwifery, 38*(4), 236–240.

Garland, N. T., & Marchione, J. (1982). A framework for analyzing the role of the NP. *Advances in Nursing Science, 4*(2), 19–20.

Hafferty, F. W., & Goldberg, H. I. (1986). Educational strategies for targeted retention of nonphysician health care providers. *Health Services Research, 2*(1), 107–125.

Hupcey, J. E. (1994). Graduate education for nurse practitioners: Are advanced degrees needed for practice? *Journal of Professional Nursing, 10*(6), 350–356.

Hupcey, J. E. (1990). The socialization process of master's level NP students. *Journal of Nursing Education, 29*(5), 196–201.

Jones, N. E. (1992). Injury prevention: A survey of clinical practice. *Journal of Pediatric Health Care, 6*, 182–186.

Koch, L. W., Pazaki, S. H., & Campbell, J. D. (1992). The first 20 years of nurse practitioner literature: An evolution of joint practice issues. *Nurse Practitioner, 17*(2), 62–71.

Lange, L., Haak, S., Lincoln, M., Thompson, C., Turner, C., Weir, C., Foerster, V., Nilasena, D., & Reeves, R. (1997). Use of Iliad to improve diagnostic performance of nurse practitioner students. *Journal of Nursing Education, 36*(1), 36–45.

Lindeke, L., Canedy, B., & Kay, M. (1997). A comparison of practice domains of clinical nurse specialists and nurse practitioners. *Journal of Professional Nursing, 13*(5), 281–287.

McCaig, L., Hooker, R., Sekscenski, E., & Woodwell, D. (1998). Physical assistance and NPs in hospital outpatient departments. *Public Health Reports, 118,* 75–82.

Morgan, W. A., & Trolinger, J. (1994). The clinical education of primary care NP students. *The Nurse Practitioner, 19*(4), 62–66.

Murdock, J. E., & Neafsey, P. J. (1995). Self efficacy measurements: An approach for predicting practice outcomes in continuing education? *The Journal of Continuing Education in Nursing, 26*(4), 158–165.

National Organization of Nurse Practitioner Faculties. (1995). *Advanced nursing practice: Curriculum guidelines and program standards for nurse practitioner education.* Washington, DC: National Organization of Nurse Practitioner Faculties.

Office of Technology Assessment. (1986). Nurse practitioners, physician assistants, and certified nurse midwives: A policy analysis. (Health Technology Case Study No. 37). Washington, DC: U.S. Government Printing Office.

Pew Health Professions Commission. (1991). Healthy America: Practitioners for 2005. An agenda for action for U.S. health professional schools. Durham, NC: Duke University Press.

Rasch, R. S., & Frauman, A. (1996). Advanced practice in nursing: Conceptual issues. *Journal of Professional Nursing, 12*(3), 141–146.

Rolfe, G., & Phillips, L. (1997). The development and evaluation of the role of an advanced nurse practitioner in dementia—an action research project. *International Journal of Nursing Studies, 34*(2), 119–127.

Sackett, D. L., Spitzer, W. O., Gent, M., & Roberts, R. S. (1974). The Burlington randomized trial of the nurse practitioner: Health outcomes of patients. *Annals of Internal Medicine, 80,* 137–142.

Safriet, B. J. (1992). Health care dollars and regulatory sense: The role of advanced practice nursing. *Yale Journal of Regulation, 9*(2), 417–488.

Shah, H., Bruttomesso, K., Sullivan, D., & Lattanzio, J. (1997). An evaluation of the role and practices of the acute-care nurse practitioner. *AACN Clinical Issues, 8*(1), 147–155.

Shah, H. S., Sullivan, D. T., Lattanzio, J., & Bruttomesso, K. M. (1993). Standards for educational programs: Preparing students as acute care nurse practitioners. *American Association of Critical Care Nurses Clinical Issues, 4*(4), 593–598.

Spitzer, W. O., Sackett, D. L., Sibley, J. C., Roberts, R. S., Tech, M., Gent, M., Kergin, D. J., Hackett, B. C., & Olynich, A. (1974). The Burlington randomized trial of the nurse practitioner. *New England Journal of Medicine, 290,* 251–256.

Swingler, G. H. (1994). An evaluation of a board game as an aid to reach neonatal primary care. *Curationis, 17*(1), 38–39.

Talashek, M. I., Gerace, L. M., Miller, A. G., & Lindsey, M. (1995). Family nurse practitioner clinical competencies in alcohol and substance abuse. *Journal of the American Academy of Nurse Practitioners, 7*(2), 57–63.

Thibodeau, J. A., & Hawkins, J. W. (1994). Moving toward a nursing model in advanced practice. *Western Journal of Nursing Research, 16*(2), 205–218.

Walsh, L. V., & Jaspan, A. L. (1990). Lay midwife to nurse-midwife: Perceived learning needs and attitudes toward the learning experience. *Journal of Nurse-Midwifery, 35*(4), 204–213.

Wilbur, J., Zoeller, L. H., Talashek, M. I., & Sullivan, J. A. (1990). Career trends of master's prepared family nurse practitioners. *Journal of the American Academy of Nurse Practitioners, 2*(2), 69–78.

Chapter 7

Utilization of Master's and Doctoral Program Graduates: Implications for Curricula— 1999 Update

BETSY FRANK, RN, PHD

INTRODUCTION

The American health care system is in a dramatic period of change. More health care is being delivered in interdisciplinary managed care settings. Furthermore, the percentage of elderly seeking health care continues to increase.

Through the Nursing's Agenda for Health Care Reform (American Nurses Association [ANA], 1992), the ANA stated that all nurses, especially those with postbaccalaureate degrees, should and can have a central role in the restructured system. The Institute of Medicine supports this notion, stating that hospitals should expand their use of advanced-practice nurses in order to provide clinical leadership and to help manage complex patients in a cost-efficient manner (Wunderlich, Sloan, & Davis, 1996). The 1995 Pew Commission Report recommended that the numbers of master's-level nurse practitioner programs be increased (Pew Health Professions Commission, 1995).

The history of master's and doctoral education has been well documented (Brown, 1978; Hudacek & Carpenter, 1994). However, there is a need to assess current utilization of nurses with graduate degrees, and their future needs, to help educators plan for curricula that meet the demands of the turbulent health care environment.

In order to evaluate utilization of and demand for nurses with advanced degrees, both Medline and the Cumulative Index to Nursing and Allied Health Literature (CINAHL) were searched via on-line and CD-ROM methods. For the first edition of this chapter (Frank, 1996), the years 1978 to 1992 were searched in Medline using the descriptors "master's and doctoral programs." These same descriptors were used for the 1983–1994 CINAHL search. This update added a CINAHL search of research articles, dissertation abstracts, and full text sources for 1994 to 1998. Older articles were located through bibliographic references cited in retrieved information. Additionally, a CINAHL search was conducted using the descriptors "graduate nursing education/evaluation." This limited search yielded 105 references for the years 1982 to 1998, not all of which were pertinent. Finally, since nurse practitioners and clinical nurse specialists play integral roles in a reformed health care system, a CD-ROM Medline search using the years 1990 to 1994 was conducted for the first edition of the chapter using the "nurse practitioner" and "clinical nurse specialist" role descriptor terms. The Medline search was not updated for this revised chapter, because research for the first edition revealed that most of the Medline references were also located through the CINAHL search.

One problem encountered during the literature search for the first edition was that national data sets which described the utilization of advanced-practice nurses, including those with graduate degrees, were often contained in government documents not printed by the U.S. Government Printing Office. These printed sources had to be located through private organizations such as the Indiana State Nurses Association. A summary of more current data sets, however, is now located on-line via the World Wide Web. (See, for example, http://158.72.83.3/bhpr/dn/sampsrv.htm.) Once the on-line summary is located, the researcher has a contact point to obtain a full report of the summary data presented.

Guided by national data sets, articles were placed into the categories of current employment patterns, general role preparation, and specific role preparation. Tables found throughout this chapter summarize the literature reviewed.

CURRENT EMPLOYMENT PATTERNS

According to the Health Resources and Services Administration, Bureau of Health Professions (1997), an estimated 193,159 or 9.1% of registered nurses have their master's degree in nursing or a related field. This is an increase of 1.6% over the 1994 figures (Health Resources and Services Administration, 1994a). Master's-prepared nurses function as educators, administrators, and advanced-practice clinicians (see Table 7–1).

The Health Resources and Services Administration (1997) also estimates that 14,300 employed nurses have doctoral degrees in nursing or a related field (an increase of 3,000 over 1994). Approximately 58% are employed in education or research positions, and an additional 24% list their employment as primarily administrator or assistant (Health Resources and Services Administration, 1997). The majority of doctorally prepared educators work in baccalaureate and higher degree programs (personal communication, August 28, 1997, National League for Nursing). These figures have not changed much from research conducted in the early 1980s. At that time, a survey of the entire population of doctorally prepared nurses revealed that 76% of the 1,964 respondents worked in academic institutions (Brimmer et al., 1983) (Table 7–2).

TABLE 7–1.
Numbers of Employed Master's- and Doctorally-Prepared Nurses

Practice Focus	Master's Degree	Doctoral Degree
Total	193,159[a]	14,300[a]
Clinical practice	86,758[a, b]	1,737[a]
Education	31,206[a, c]	7,749[a, c]
Research	2,033[a]	493[a]
Administration	48,337[a, c]	3,753[a, c]
Other	24,842[d]	568[d]

[a]Health Resources and Services Administration (1997).
[b]Includes all advanced nurse practitioners and other clinical positions.
[c]Includes academic and service positions.
[d]Includes all other positions including consultants and undefined categories.

TABLE 7–2.
Current Employment Patterns

Author/Date	Sample	Method	Findings
Brimmer (1983)	1,964 RNs with doctorates.	Investigator-designed survey.	Most employed in baccalaureate and higher degree programs.
Health Resources & Services Administration (1994a)	National sample survey.	Differential state sampling—investigator designed.	Reports 50 state employment patterns as national aggregate data.
Health Resources & Services Administration (1997)	National sample survey.	Differential state sampling—investigator designed.	Reports 50 state employment patterns as national aggregate data.

GENERAL ROLE PREPARATION

Knowing what is expected of those who have completed graduate programs in nursing helps faculty to plan and implement appropriate curricula. The only studies found concerning general role preparation dealt exclusively with master's graduates (see Table 7–3). Studies outlining expectations of doctoral program graduates concerned preparation for the educator and researcher roles only.

An early study delineated essential competencies for master's-prepared nurses (McLane, 1978). From a thorough literature review, a reliable and valid questionnaire was developed. A large random sample of deans, directors of graduate programs, and selected students from each program lent much credibility to the study's findings, but the number of respondents in each subgroup was not identified. All respondents designated 25 items on the questionnaire as core competencies. McLane classified the core competencies into interpersonal, research, accountability, change agent, educator, and humanizer categories. Although this study was reported 20 years ago, many of the expected competencies remain today.

Hill (1989) conducted a needs assessment for the purpose of planning a new master's program. Although not explicitly describing the sample, Hill implied that all registered nurses within a 60-mile radius of the university who held a baccalaureate degree or higher were surveyed, resulting in a responding sample size of 47. Statements from a previous Delphi survey were used to construct a questionnaire

TABLE 7–3.
General Role Preparation

Author/Date	Sample	Method	Findings
Burns et al. (1993)	175 master's programs.	Descriptive, investigator-designed instrument.	Curricula designed around multiple specialties and functional areas.
Frauman & Germino (1998)	153 nephrology nurses.	Descriptive, investigator-designed instrument.	Interest in graduate study, but travel a problem.
Gieske (1995)	289 students in four different master's programs.	Discriminant analysis of predictor variables.	Combination of academic and demographic variables best predicts success.
Hansen & Pozehl (1995)	59 master's graduates.	Ex post facto, GPRS visual analogue scale (measures cognitive ability).	Nonnursing GPA and GRE verbal score predicted score on GPRS.
Heller et al. (1989)	128 nursing directors, 188 generic BSN, 74 RN BSN, 315 staff nurses, 30 journal readers	Descriptive, investigator-designed survey.	Strong interest expressed for informatics skills.
Hill (1989)	13 administrators, 34 staff nurses.	Descriptive, investigator-designed survey.	Interdisciplinary program recommended.
Hungler et al. (1979)	272 master's graduates.	Theoretically based, investigator-designed survey.	Educators scored higher on measures of professionalism.

TABLE 7–3.
General Role Preparation (Continued)

Author/Date	Sample	Method	Findings
McLane (1978)	133 deans, directors of nursing, and graduate students.	Investigator-designed survey.	25 core competencies identified.
O'Sullivan et al. (1997)	237 BSN programs, 91 master's programs.	Descriptive investigator-designed survey.	15% had collected aggregate data, 22% had definition of critical thinking.
Ryan & Carlton (1997)	One program.	Program evaluation model.	Portfolio to document outcomes.
Smith (1980)	37 graduates, 20 employers.	Investigator-designed program evaluation.	Useful coursework and skills described. Areas for improvement identified.

BSN = bachelor of science in nursing
GPA = grade point average
GPRS = graduate performance rating scale
GRE = graduate record exam
RN = registered nurse

containing 18 predictive statements concerning the health care system in the year 2000. Participants estimated the probability of occurrence for each statement and suggested program content areas. Based on survey results and the higher education climate in the state, the author recommended starting an interdisciplinary master's program with content in leadership, communication, counseling, and nursing theory. As recommended by study participants, master's-level gerontology content was not included. Considering the changing demographics in the United States, this advice is somewhat perplexing. However, working within interdisciplinary environments is a requirement of all nurses with graduate degrees. Therefore, all nursing faculty might consider ways to provide interdisciplinary experiences for students, while at the same time incorporating opportunities to explore the richness of advanced nursing knowledge.

Surveys have also identified needs for specialty education. For example, Frauman and Germino (1998) surveyed members of the American Nephrology Nurses' Association in three southern states. They found that nurses were interested in specialty preparation at the master's level, but travel to the university location made future enrollment unlikely.

One particular skill not identified by McLane or Hill was competency with informatics. Heller, Damrosch, Romano, and McCarthy (1989) assessed the need for a master's program with an emphasis on informatics as applied to the field of nursing. A regional sample of nurse executives, students, and staff nurses from selected academic/research hospitals, and readers of a 1987 issue of *Computers in Nursing* ($N = 735$), were surveyed regarding their perceived need for and interest in a master's program with an informatics specialty. Survey results and letters of endorsement led to curriculum planning. Since the 1980s the question has become not whether to include informatics content in master's programs but how much and what kind of content should be included.

Specific needs assessments, whether on a national or a local level, are useful in curriculum planning. Knowing what already exists in master's education nationwide can give faculty more information upon which to support decisions regarding curricula. Burns et al. (1993) provided a useful database for faculty. These researchers sought to determine program admission requirements and curricular organization by examining written documents sent to prospective students. More than 99% of the 176 master's programs responded to the mail survey. Results indicated that required semester credit hours ranged from 29 to 59 with a mean of 36 hours of credit. Eighty-eight percent required a bachelor of science–nursing (BSN) for admission and most required a 3.0 grade point average (GPA) and at least one year of clinical practice. Only 4% required computer literacy for admission. More than 50% also required some preadmission standardized test, such as the Graduate Records Exam (GRE). Burns et al. concluded that multiple models existed for master's education and no consensus was present for functional role preparation for administrators or educators. They also noted that the nature of the expected research competency for master's graduates was less than clear from the written materials. Identified gaps in curricula included lack of coursework on health policy. An additional recommendation was that the American Association of Colleges of Nursing (AACN) should develop a document regarding essential content and skills for master's education. Such a document has since been developed (AACN, 1996).

Current accreditation requirements from regional and professional accrediting bodies focus on program outcomes such as graduation rates, demonstration of particular abilities such as critical thinking, and employer satisfaction with graduates. Published data regarding the required criteria, however, are somewhat sparse.

O'Sullivan, Blevins-Stephens, Smith, and Vaughn-Wrobel (1997) surveyed 628 National League for Nursing (NLN)–accredited baccalaureate and higher degree programs to discover how programs measured the critical thinking outcome. Over 34% of master's programs responded. Although the outcome-oriented approach was adopted by the NLN in 1991, as of 1994 few master's programs had decided how to measure this outcome criteria. While critical thinking is a worthy outcome, perhaps its precise definition and measurement are problematic.

Ryan and Carlton (1997) proposed a model to measure a variety of cognitive outcomes through a portfolio method. While no outcome data were presented, their model appears to have potential for collating these outcomes of graduate education.

Another way to look at outcomes of graduate education is to analyze which students are likely to complete educational programs. Two studies explored student characteristics that predicted educational success (Gieske, 1995; Hansen & Pozehl, 1995). Gieske (1995), in a study of 289 graduate students, found that a combination of demographic and academic variables best predicts graduation from a master's program. In fact, her discriminate analysis showed that gender, age, race, and hours worked outside of school were weighted more heavily than undergraduate GPA and GRE scores. A problem with her study, however, was that her data were collected 11 to 15 years prior to publication. One wonders if changing student demographics would have altered her findings.

Hansen and Pozehl (1995) investigated actual performance in a master's program as opposed to simply completion of the program. They analyzed the relationship between admission criteria and performance on the Graduate Performance Rating Scale (GPRS), a visual analog instrument that measured communication skills, creativity, motivation, explanatory/reasoning capabilities, and other behaviors expected of master's graduates. Faculty raters familiar with the students used student records of these behaviors to judge the 59 students in the sample. Results supported the use of undergraduate nonnursing GPA and GRE scores, particularly the verbal component, as significant predictors of success. The nonnursing undergraduate GPA was a predictor of the explanatory/reasoning and synthesis scales on the GPRS. In addition, there was a low correlation between the graduate GPA and the total score on the GPRS. The authors suggested that the GPRS may be a more sensitive measure of outcomes than GPA, as it measures the expected behaviors of master's program graduates.

Another measure of effectiveness of an educational program is the degree to which role socialization occurs. Busen and Jones (1995) evaluated the leadership potential of 21 pediatric nurse practitioner graduates. As part of their study, they measured personality characteristics using the Myers–Briggs Personality Inventory, the Kolb Learning Style Inventory, and the Hoffmeister's Self-Esteem Questionnaire. Leadership potential was measured via the Conflict Mode Instrument and the Hall and Williams Change Agent Questionnaire. Results revealed that graduates showed no change in ability to handle conflict or function as a change agent when compared to their abilities at entrance in the program, and there was no significant relationship between leadership abilities and personality characteristics. The learning styles of the graduates were predominantly concrete. Thus, the authors concluded that dealing with change, management, and leadership theories was often difficult. Given that leadership behaviors are expected of master's program graduates, faculty may want to make a concerted effort to include opportunities for practicing such behaviors during the educational program.

Surveys of graduates and employers are a common way to evaluate the use and effectiveness of graduates. However, only two rather old studies were found that reported graduates' and employers' evaluation of the general role performance of master's graduates (Hungler, Krawczyk, Joyce, & Polit, 1979; Smith, 1980).

Hungler et al. (1979) discovered that those in the educator role displayed more professional behaviors than did clinicians. Hungler et al. speculated that more incentives for professional behaviors existed for educators, and the authors encouraged faculty to investigate ways to increase professional behaviors for all graduates. Their advice seems quite timely almost 20 years later.

Smith's (1980) findings seemed to corroborate those of Hungler et al. (1979). She found that employers rated graduates' leadership behaviors somewhat lower than did the graduates themselves. One particular strength of this study was its inclusion of the survey instrument, which could be used in other follow-up studies of master's graduates.

Nurse Practitioners and Clinical Nurse Specialists

The focus of the aforementioned studies was general. Utilization and effectiveness issues may also be analyzed by examining specific roles within which graduates function to identify strengths, weaknesses, and gaps in current curricular models. Table 7–4 summarizes literature regarding specific role preparation for advanced clinical practice roles.

A recent national survey estimated that 110,900 nurses were certified and employed as nurse practitioners (NPs) or clinical nurse specialists (CNSs), nurse clinicians, or nurse midwives (Health Resources and Services Administration, 1997). Only 61.9% of NPs and midwives (whose numbers were combined) were master's prepared, while almost 42% of CNSs and 13% of nurse clinicians were prepared as such. One might expect the number of NPs with master's degrees to rise as certification requirements change to require master's preparation, and in fact because the 1992 survey (published in 1994) showed that 40% of NPs were master's prepared (Health Resources and Services Administration, 1994a). A 1992 survey also showed a greater proportion of CNSs who were master's prepared, but the 1997 data appear to have a larger total estimate of persons functioning in this job category as compared to the 1992 data, perhaps due to a different sampling methods or the fact that many master's-prepared clinicians are employed in schools of nursing. The majority of the certified practitioners (31%) were prepared exclusively as family nurse practitioners, and 36% were prepared as adult health and pediatric nurse practitioners. Survey participants identified a multiplicity of specific practice settings and clinical foci.

In addition to the published statistics from the federal government, data are also available from individual states. For example, Tennessee, North Carolina, and Louisiana have conducted studies of advanced-practice nurses including nurse practitioners (Cannon & Beare, 1997; Johnson, 1996; Smith, Moody,

TABLE 7–4.
*Nurse Practitioners, Clinical Nurse Specialists,
& Other Advanced Nurse Practitioners*

Author/Date	Sample	Method	Findings
Bachman (1995)	191 school nurses.	Descriptive survey, investigator designed.	70% interested in MSN program.
Baradell (1994)	Not applicable.	Literature review.	Demonstrated cost effectiveness of CNSs.
Barkauskas & Blaha (1989)	98 master's programs.	Investigator-designed survey.	32 programs considering home care majors or courses.
Beal et al. (1996)	258 NNPs.	Descriptive, correlational.	Most NNPs certificate prepared. Master's-prepared NNPs were more nursing oriented.
Brophy et al. (1989)	23 hospitals.	Investigator-designed interview and written survey.	CNSs have administrative duties and need broad range of theory and skills.
Brown & Grimes (1995)	38 NP and 15 NM studies.	Meta-analysis.	Quality of care equivalent or better than MD.
Buchanan (1996)	1 hospital, 96 patients.	Program evaluation.	Collaborative behaviors of nurses and NPs increased.
Busen & Jones (1995)	21 PNP students.	Standardized instruments.	Most students were concrete thinkers; abstract learners had more characteristics of change agents.
Cairo (1996)	5 ER physicians.	Grounded theory.	NPs viewed as dependent collaborators.
Cannon & Beare (1997)	89 hospital administrators, 31 parish health administrators.	Survey.	Roles fulfilled by 234 master's-prepared nurses described.
Christensen et al. (1985)	73 MS-prepared OHNs.	Investigator-designed survey.	OHNs participate in organizational decision making.
Caldwell et al. (1996)	71 cardiovascular CNSs.	Investigator-designed survey.	CNSs educated in traditional role and employed in hospital setting.
Chamberlin & Rogers (1997)	10 focus groups and 787 survey participants.	Investigator-designed survey and interviews.	Description of practice levels in occupational health nursing.

TABLE 7-4.
Nurse Practitioners, Clinical Nurse Specialists,
& Other Advanced Nurse Practitioners (Continued)

Author/Date	Sample	Method	Findings
Chase et al. (1996)	66 CNSs and NPs from one hospital and one contact from each of 10 hospitals.	Investigator-designed survey.	Some role confusion, which resulted in retitling of those in advanced-practice roles.
Derstine (1992)	18 rehabilitation CNS graduates, 5 employers.	Telephone and mail investigator-designed survey.	Only 3 graduates functioned as CNSs; others used knowledge in broader context. Employers said graduates met program objectives.
Dunn (1993a, 1993b)	Random sample of 800 NAPNAP members (520 responded).	Investigator-designed survey.	38.5% have MS degree. Members are meeting primary health care needs of children in underserved areas.
Elder & Bullough (1990)	28 CNS graduates, 46 NP graduates.	Investigator-designed survey based on literature and practice patterns.	Both groups function in similar ways.
Fenton (1992)	34 MS RNs.	Ethnographic.	8 work role competencies explained.
Fenton & Brykczynski (1993)	242 CNS clinical situations, 199 NP clinical situations.	Secondary analysis of qualitative data.	NPs have one added domain of practice; other domains similar.
Forbes et al. (1990)	108 master's programs.	Investigator-designed survey.	NP and CNS programs are more alike than different.
Froerer (1998)	61 advanced-practice nurses.	Investigator-designed survey.	Lack of adequate training a barrier to inclusion of endoscopy on practice modalities.
Gallagher et al. (1992)	153 oncology CNSs, 144 oncology CNSs.	Two-round Delphi.	Clinical focus an important part of practice.
Guzik et al. (1992)	65 OHNs.	Investigator-designed survey; descriptive correlational.	Internal consultants provide more direct care. External consultants have more administrative tasks.
Haw (1996)	108 schools of nursing.	Investigator-designed instrument.	At least 8 schools with graduate programs in case management.

TABLE 7–4.
Nurse Practitioners, Clinical Nurse Specialists,
& Other Advanced Nurse Practitioners (Continued)

Author/Date	Sample	Method	Findings
Health Resources and Services Administration (1990)	National databases.	Projection of supply and demand.	Outlined projected needs for advanced nurse practitioners.
Ingersoll (1995)	35 acute care advanced-practice nurses.	Semistructured interviews.	Positive patient care outcomes not precisely defined.
Jacobs et al. (1998)	259 RNs.	Investigator-designed questionnaire.	43% of continence nurses were master's prepared. Lack of understanding of role and reimbursement were barriers to practice.
Johnson (1996)	73,000 North Carolina RNs.	Investigator-designed survey.	3% were advanced-practice nurses.
Journal of the American Academy of Nurse Practitioners (1994)	75 graduate programs.	Investigator-designed survey.	61 offer post-master's NP certificate programs.
Kinney et al. (1997)	129 NPs employed in oncology.	Investigator-designed semistructured questionnaire.	Description of role functions of NPs in oncology settings.
Kleinpell (1997)	126 applicants for ACNP certification exam.	Modified previously used survey instrument.	Description of work setting and roles of ACNPs.
Lindeke et al. (1997)	15 postmaster's NPs.	Qualitative.	CNS and NP roles viewed as distinct.
Louis & Sabo (1994)	68 nurse administrators, 42 NPs, 323 MDs.	Investigator-designed survey based on State Board of Nursing protocols.	49.7% willing to hire NPs. NP group most likely to hire and MD group least likely.
Mahoney (1994)	373 MDs, 296 NPs.	Clinical judgment of case vignettes.	NPs displayed more appropriate practice decisions.
McGovern et al. (1985)	73 OHNs.	Investigator-designed survey.	77% employed in occupational health settings; engaged in management, teaching, and direct care roles.

TABLE 7-4.
Nurse Practitioners, Clinical Nurse Specialists,
& Other Advanced Nurse Practitioners (Continued)

Author/Date	Sample	Method	Findings
Melkus & Fain (1995)	172 NPs.	Investigator-designed instrument.	Description of NP practice patterns relative to diabetes care. Based on data, diabetes concentration added to master's program.
Pitts & Seimer (1998)	42 CNOs of pediatric hospitals.	Investigator-designed survey.	50% hospitals require MS for NP role.
Radke et al. (1990)	46 CNS graduates.	Investigator-designed survey.	CNSs participate in a variety of administrative tasks.
Ramsey et al. (1993)	101 patients.	Investigator-designed survey.	Patients very satisfied with care.
Ruth-Sanchez et al. (1996)	673 NNPs.	Investigator-designed survey.	39% master's prepared. All more facilitated than constrained in practice.
Segall & McKay (1984)	43 community health graduates.	Investigator-designed survey.	Aggregate-based learning very useful. Graduates wanted more administrative content.
Selby et al. (1991)	588 community health nursing leaders from a national sample.	Investigator-designed survey based upon NLN and ACHNE criteria.	Core content included administration, epidemiology, community health assessment.
Smith et al. (1996)	54 NPs in Tennessee.	Investigator adaptation of standardized survey.	Demographic characteristics and practice patterns described.
Stokes et al. (1997)	85 master's programs.	Investigator-designed survey.	Conrad and Pratt model described environmental and curricular variables.
Towers (1989, 1990)	5,964 NPs from a national sample.	Investigator-designed survey.	50% FNPs were master's prepared, compared with 24.8% of women's health NPs.
Whitfill & Burst (1994)	40 CNM programs.	Program description survey.	Majority of CNM programs are contained within MS programs.

TABLE 7–4.
Nurse Practitioners, Clinical Nurse Specialists,
& Other Advanced Nurse Practitioners (Continued)

Author/Date	Sample	Method	Findings
Wills & Delahoussaye (1998)	50 graduate programs.	Investigator-designed survey.	Program description of 43 schools offering home health content.
Wood et al. (1996)	1,061 California CNSs.	Investigator-designed survey.	65% master's prepared. Specialty areas and role components described.

ACHNE = Association of Community Health Nursing Educators
ACNP = acute care nurse practitioner
CNM = certified nurse midwife
CNO = chief nursing officer
ER = emergency room
FNP = family nurse practitioner
MD = medical doctor
MS = master of science
MSN = master of science–nursing
NAPNAP = National Association of Pediatric Nurse Practitioners
NLN = National League for Nursing
NM = nurse midwife
NNP = neonatal nurse practitioner
NP = nurse practitioner
OHN = occupational health nurse
PNP = pediatric nurse practitioner
RN = registered nurse

Glenn, & Garmany, 1996). State studies are aimed at determining geographical distribution of practitioners and functions they perform in the states' health care delivery systems. These studies are particularly useful to those in the states in question who are planning new graduate programs or revising current programs.

Primary care is one cornerstone of health care reform. Nurse practitioners have a vital role to play in providing primary health care services. Knowing how practitioners are used will help nurse educators to plan appropriate educational programs.

Towers (1989) surveyed 12,000 members of the American Academy of Nurse Practitioners. Almost 50% responded, which is sufficient to evaluate national employment trends. Those with master's degrees ranged from 52.5% for family nurse practitioners to 24.8% for women's health practitioners. More than three-fourths of psychiatric specialists had master's degrees. The majority worked in urban areas, and almost one quarter had hospital admitting privileges (Towers, 1990).

Dunn (1993b) reported a national study of pediatric nurse practitioners (PNPs) who were members of the National Association of Pediatric Nurse Practitioners (NAPNAP). In 1992, 38.5% of those surveyed had been prepared at the master's level as compared with 17% in 1977 (Dunn, 1993a). Regardless of educational preparation, PNPs were providing independent primary care to children in a variety of settings. Most often these children were from low socioeconomic groups (Dunn, 1993b). Thus, data indicate that nurse practitioners are meeting the health care needs of underserved groups.

A more recent study (Pitts & Seimer, 1998) of tertiary care children's hospitals showed that 50% of hospitals surveyed required a master's degree for persons practicing as PNPs. Most PNPs worked with protocols and functioned collaboratively with physicians, and the majority worked in specialty areas, which might be expected in such settings.

The pediatric inpatient arena is not the only place where nurse practitioners are being utilized. A current trend is employment of NPs in a variety of acute care settings including the neonatal intensive care unit and adult critical care units.

Beal, Maguire, and Carr (1996) conducted a study to determine the identity of neonatal nurse practitioners (NNPs) as advanced-practice nurses. One finding of note was that nurses prepared at the master's level, as opposed to those prepared at the certificate level, had more identity with the nursing profession. Certainly this finding gives credence to the notion that master's-prepared nurse practitioners are not merely physician extenders but nurses practicing at an advanced level.

Ruth-Sanchez, Lee, and Bosque (1996) conducted a study of practice patterns of NNPs. Using a national data set similar to Beal et al.'s (1995), Ruth-Sanchez et al. found that the majority of NNPs were prepared at the certificate level. The majority (48%) of NNPs reported to medical supervisors and 33% to nursing supervisors, and the remaining subjects reported to both. Most were satisfied with their jobs, and facilitators for job satisfaction included family satisfaction with care delivered. The authors expressed concern that despite overall job satisfaction of the NNPs, control of this advanced nursing practice role outside of nursing was problematic. Given that the majority of NNPs are not master's prepared and might not identify with nursing per se, this concern seems valid.

During the past four years, more reports have appeared in the literature with regard to the role of the acute care nurse practitioner. This advanced-practice nurse often works in critical units or multispecialty clinics in tertiary care or community hospitals. Ingersoll (1995), evaluating the role of master's-prepared acute nurse practitioners who worked in major medical centers, found that they described their roles as complementary to physicians. These advanced-practice nurses were seen as practitioners who could affect patient outcomes in a positive, but undefined, manner. In addition to direct care given, they worked with staff nurses to establish protocols for patient care. Based on these findings, the author recommended that acute care practitioners begin to document more precisely their role in and effect on patient care.

Buchanan (1996) accomplished such documentation in an evaluation study of acute nurse practitioners in a collaborative practice with physicians. Clinical logs were kept that documented how the practitioners spent their time, data were collected that documented characteristics of patients cared for. Since the data were obtained as a part of introducing a new role to a patient care area, before and after data were collected with regard to perception of collaborative practice. Although physicians did not sense more collaborative relationships, nurses and nurse practitioners did. Perhaps the nurses supported the new role more than did the physicians. Another important finding was that the nurse practitioners cared for more of the elderly, female, chronically ill patients. This confirms the notion that advanced-practice nursing curricula need to capitalize on their strength in preparing students to care for the elderly.

Kleinpell (1997) surveyed master's-prepared acute care nurse practitioners who were the first to take the certification exam for this specialty practice domain. Many of the practitioners had new positions created for them, in which they performed invasive procedures, such as chest tube insertion, traditionally reserved for medical staff. Although specific data were not presented to confirm this conclusion, Kleinpell stated that the practitioners did much more than these medical tasks and did integrate the advanced nursing role with the medical aspects of their jobs. If this conclusion is indeed valid, the importance of master's preparation for advanced roles is further verified.

In addition to general acute care nurse practitioner roles, advanced-practice nurses function in specialty practitioner roles that may be an "add-on" to their certification areas. For example, nurse practitioners may work in oncology. Kinney, Hawkins, and Hudman (1997) surveyed 266 nurse practitioners who were members of the Oncology Nurses Society. Over 80% of the 129 who responded were master's or doctorally prepared, and their nurse practitioner certification was in a variety of fields including family, adult, and women's health. Like other authors, Kinney et al. found that the advanced nurse practitioners had melded their nursing roles with traditional medical roles, but the nursing component remained paramount in their practice.

Although not acute care focused, currently another add-on role is that of the school nurse practitioner. Bachman (1995) surveyed school nurses to determine what practitioner specialties were appropriate in the school health setting. Twenty-nine percent of respondents identified the need for a specific school health focus, but the others identified family and pediatric practitioner preparation as valuable. Since many of the school nurses were not even baccalaureate prepared, the author recommended that educators consider registered nurse (RN) to master of science in nursing (MSN) programs for this population. She also recommended that the programs be offered part time and via distance education to accommodate the working nurse not located near a university campus. Bachman noted that her own university, Barnes College of Nursing at the University of Missouri–St. Louis, was using her findings in its program planning.

Knowing how current practitioners are used is important because this information can be used to justify program design, including clinical practicums contained therein. Yet equally important for future planning is employers' willingness to use graduates from nurse practitioner programs. Louis and Sabo (1994) investigated disposition to hire nurse practitioners in Nevada. Study participants included nurse practitioners, nurse executives, and physicians. Less than 25% of mailed surveys were returned; only 43% of physicians had had experience with practitioners. 71% of physicians and 42% of nursing administrators saw a need for NPs, and 26% of physicians said they would not hire NPs even though they had had experience with them. Respondents most frequently cited the need for family and gerontological nurse practitioners. Physicians and others with baccalaureate and higher university degrees saw less need for NPs than did those with diplomas and associate degrees. The authors wondered if responses would have been different if a master's degree had been required of all NPs, as was not the case. Not knowing the scope of practice for NPs may have been a problem for the survey respondents. One of the major recommendations of the study was to disseminate more information regarding nurse practitioners.

In a more recent study, Cairo (1996) interviewed five board-certified emergency room physicians who worked in emergency rooms where no nurse practitioners were employed. Two of the physicians had prior experience working with nurse practitioners and three didn't. The findings of this qualitative study revealed that physicians viewed the nurse practitioner role as a somewhat dependent, yet collaborative role. Physicians were concerned that NPs would substitute for physicians rather than practice advanced-practice nursing. This concern points to the fact that educators and practitioners need to work with the medical community to help its members better understand the role of nurse practitioners. The student practicum experience may be a place where this could occur. If this educational effort is not successful, new graduates may not be able to find jobs that match their capabilities.

What seems clear, then, is that faculty who are planning nurse practitioner programs need to meet with potential employers and help them understand the role of the nurse practitioner. Reticence to use nurse practitioners may be related to lack of knowledge about the role.

Advanced-practice nurses also function in traditional clinical specialist roles. While this role is not a new advanced-practice role, there is still some confusion regarding its function. Traditionally, those who are clinical nurse specialists are educated to provide direct care, educate health care staff and students, participate in research, and perform some administrative functions (Chase, Johnson, Laffoon, Jacobs, & Johnson, 1996). Many who claim the title of clinical specialist are not master's prepared. Chase et al. (1996) found from a survey of 10 hospitals that 70% required those claiming the title of clinical specialist to have a master's degree; this is despite the fact that a master's degree is required for certification. A statewide survey of nurses in California found that only 65% of clinical specialists were master's prepared (Wood, Caldwell, Cusack, Claar-Rice, & Dibble, 1996). As with nurse practitioners, titles held do not always reflect graduate school preparation.

Assessing the specific need and utilization for clinical specialists was frequently reported by specialty area of practice. A plethora of specialty foci, primarily in the adult health area, seems to exist (Stokes, Whitis, & Moore-Thrasher, 1997).

Segall and McKay (1984) surveyed community health graduates from one school in Colorado and their supervisors, and Selby, Riportella-Muller, Salmon, Lagault, and Quade (1991) sampled community health nursing leaders nationwide.[1] Segall and McKay (1984) found that 46% of the graduates were employed in education, 39% in administration, and 15% in clinical practice. Graduates rated clinical content as the most useful and functional role content the least beneficial. The authors attributed this finding to the fact that graduates may have had an increased demand for advanced clinical knowledge. Graduates saw the need, however, for additional content in administration. Respondents and their supervisors validated success in the job environment.

Selby et al.'s (1991) more recent survey of community health nursing educational needs supported Segall and McKay's (1984) finding that administration and management should be included in community health programs, because community health leaders deemed the administrator–manager role the most important. Direct care roles and beginning competency in teaching were next in order. A majority also identified the importance of the researcher and consultant roles. The investigators discovered that while the administration–management role was critical, less than 30% of the master's programs required beginning competency in this area. The researcher role was the only listed educational competency that exceeded practice requirements. Given practice requirements, the authors recommended that faculty examine the nature of nursing core courses required of community health graduates. They also recommended that more emphasis be placed on epidemiological theories. Faculty who teach in community health majors may want to enhance adminis-

---

[1] Some authors currently do not include community health/public health nurses in the category of advanced nurse practitioners that includes clinical specialists and nurse practitioners (Cronenwett, 1995). However, federal data sets would include this specialization under the rubric of clinical practice if such nurses did not serve in an administrative capacity.

trative role content and explore what research competencies are required in contradistinction to requirements at the doctoral level.

Included in the plans for health care reform is health care offered at the work site, an effort to which occupational health nurses will be critical. Two nationwide surveys delineated the roles for master's-prepared occupational health nurses (Christensen, Richard, Froberg, McGovern, & Abanobi, 1985; Guzik, McGovern, & Kochervar, 1992; McGovern, Richard, Christensen, Froberg, & Abanobi, 1985). Most respondents in the 1985 survey were employed in administrative positions and were actively involved in program planning and organizational decision making regardless of course preparation in these two areas. The other respondents were employed as educators and nurse practitioners (Christensen et al., 1985).

The 1992 study complemented the database regarding occupational health nurses (Guzik et al., 1992). This study described the roles of master's-prepared nurses who functioned as both consultants within an employer's firm and consultants with companies external to one employer agency. Over three-fourths of the graduates from 10 different schools were actually employed as occupational health nurses in a variety of for-profit and nonprofit agencies. Using data from a previous survey (Christensen et al., 1985), the authors estimated that 89% of those master's prepared in occupational health nursing and working in the field responded to their current survey. One strength of the study was that role theory guided the selection of job satisfaction and work situation variables. The 1992 respondents were more concerned with environmental issues, an example of the type of information that could be gained through interdisciplinary coursework. More recently, Chamberlin and Rogers (1997) surveyed members of the American Association of Occupational Health Nurses and found that members acknowledged differing levels of practice in this field. Competencies identified for the advanced levels of practice were those taught in master's programs.

Home care is another critical element of the health care delivery system. Barkauskas and Blaha (1989) found no specific master's programs in home care, but nine programs offered a subspecialty in home care and 10 others offered specific courses. In 1998, Wills and Delahoussaye reported that 11 programs offered a specific home health subspecialty, but many others included home health content in other tracks including community health. Since much of future health care given to various patient populations including the elderly is likely to occur within the home, incorporating home health content in all clinical specialist tracks may be more advantageous to graduates, as opposed to creating more specific home health programs.

Mental health clinical specialists also fill important roles within the health care system. Brophy, Rankin, Butler, and Egenes (1989) found that 96% of the hospitals that responded to their survey already employed such specialists. Critical content identified for a master's program included treatment modalities, general nursing knowledge, and administration/management. Respondents perceived teaching and staff development roles to be essential for the clinical specialists. Derstine (1992) reported a follow-up study of graduates who majored in rehabilitation nursing. One year following graduation, only three of 12 graduates specifically identified themselves as rehabilitation clinical specialists. Others were in fields, such as quality assurance, where they used the rehabilitation content. Some graduates said that even though they didn't intend to be employed in rehabilitation, the content was helpful in their jobs. Employers stated that graduates were effectively using the program's content, and the employers expected graduates to solve problems, improve quality of care, and provide leadership to others. These findings seemed to support the notion that a clinical specialist curriculum helps prepare graduates for a variety of roles.

The oncology field is another area that employs clinical specialists. The Oncology Nursing Society (ONS) has been quite active in developing guidelines for master's education (Gallagher, Spross, & Powel, 1992). In preparation for the second Oncology Nurse Specialist (OCNS) conference, Gallagher et al. conducted a two-round Delphi study. Findings revealed that a clinical focus would remain important in the face of a tightened financial environment, with collaboration between clinicians and administrators essential.

While many advanced-practice nurses function in non-hospital-based settings, cardiovascular specialists seem to defy this trend. As part of a larger survey Caldwell, Wood, and Dibble (1996) analyzed a subset of data from 71 cardiovascular nurse specialists. They found that 86% had graduate degrees and functioned primarily as clinical experts. Barriers to practice included the perception that NPs were favored over clinical nurse specialists and that their role was not understood. Also, while participation in research is a usual expectation of clinical specialists, only 60% critiqued research for use in practice. These findings may point to a need to strengthen the research utilization component of graduate programs. And, given that many in the community have cardiovascular disease, encouraging roles that function outside the hospital seems warranted.

Other health subspecialties attract clinical nurse specialists. Some nurses who function in these roles gain their education in formal graduate programs and some appear to add special skills via continuing education. An example of a formal program can be found at Yale University, where a diabetic care concentration was added to the core practitioner, specialist, and midwife specialties (Melkus & Fain, 1995). The authors noted graduates' employment patterns that justified this program's existence and found that graduates had conducted research which resulted in practice-oriented publications and research presentations. These findings seem to demonstrate that advanced direct patient care is not the only outcome of master's programs that focus on clinical specialties.

Two specialties that have largely used continuing education as a means to add credentials include gastroenterology and urology. A survey of advanced-practice nurses (largely nurse practitioners) revealed that these nurses are adding technical skills such as endoscopy to their roles (Froerer, 1998). Continence nurses not only focus on technical skills but educate patients with regard to bladder training (Jacobs, Wyman, Rowell, & Smith, 1998).

One additional advanced-practice role, the case manager, is worth mentioning. This new role has emerged with the advent of managed care. Haw (1996) discovered that 8 of 108 schools that answered her survey offered a specific graduate education program for case managers. Others offered specific content at the undergraduate and graduate levels that was relevant to case management. As managed care becomes the norm for the health care system in the United States, all graduate programs may want to consider ways to incorporate case management content into their curricula. While not all graduates will function in this role, the direct patient care of all advanced-practice nurses will be influenced by the actions of case managers. Thus, the advanced-practice nurse will need to have a thorough understanding of the case manager's impact on patient care.

Collaboration with administrators is important. Acute care clinical specialists also have felt ill-prepared to deal with administration issues (Radke, McArt, Schmitt, & Walker, 1990). Radke et al. gathered data from graduates of one program regarding past, present, and future administrative duties. In graduate school, 21% had taken courses with administration content and 85% percent stated that their graduate program should have included more content in this arena. Although only 15% currently were employed in administrative positions, many others were involved in decisions regarding institutional policies that required an administrative knowledge base.

Most of the previous studies delineating requirements for advanced practice have used survey methodology. Fenton (1992) used qualitative methods guided by Benner's (1984) work to identify competencies displayed by clinical nurse specialists. Observed competencies were the helping role, administering and monitoring therapeutic interventions, management of rapidly changing situations, diagnostic and monitoring function, teaching/coaching function, quality assessment functions, and organization and work role competencies necessary to function within a bureaucracy. In addition, a consultation role was identified. Assertive clinical specialists had more effective role performance. Each competency was described in full, but the author provided no direct quotes from study participants, perhaps because this article presented a secondary data analysis of previously reported research. The author concluded that master's curricula for clinical specialists should focus on these identified competencies, which were similarly identified by participants in other studies.

Some have proposed that dimensions of the nurse practitioner and clinical specialist roles are similar. Three recent research studies (Elder & Bullough, 1990; Fenton & Brykczynski, 1993; Forbes, Rafson, Spross, & Kozlowski, 1990) as well as a recent presentation to the AACN (Cronenwett, 1995) support this contention. Forbes et al. (1990) surveyed graduate programs in the United States with clinical specialist and/or practitioner programs. Findings revealed that curricula in both kinds of programs were similar, but practitioner programs contained more physical assessment and history taking, pharmacology, nutrition, and primary care. NP graduates functioned more in primary care and CNSs were in tertiary care settings. The authors suggested that CNS and NP programs might be merged.

Elder and Bullough's (1990) survey of graduates from one nursing program and Fenton and Brykczynski's (1993) study supported the recommendation of Forbes et al. Elder and Bullough (1990) discovered that both NPs and CNSs engaged in similar activities; however, NPs did more physical exams and prescribed treatments, and CNSs participated more in staff development. Fenton and Brykczynski (1993) conducted a secondary analysis on qualitative data previously collected to compare the NP and the CNS roles. Findings from this comparative study showed that in addition to the CNS competencies previously described by Fenton (1992), NPs displayed a competency entitled "management of patient health/illness status." Further, CNSs had more role ambiguity. These authors suggested that curricula for NPs and CNSs be developed with a common core but different clinical applications.

Lindeke, Canedy, and Kay (1997), studying 15 nurse practitioners who had been previously educated as clinical nurse specialists, confirmed Fenton and Bryczynski's (1993) work. Their findings reinforced that the clinical nurse specialist role is distinct from the nurse practitioner role. It would seem, then, that educators are obliged to clarify the preparation for these roles.

Additional advanced clinical roles for master's-prepared graduates are the certified nurse anesthetist (CRNA) and certified nurse midwife (CNM). Currently, there are an estimated 7,400 CNMs, and of those 2,400 have master's degrees (Health Resources and Services Administration, 1990). The master's degree is not a requirement for midwifery certification; however, 32 of 40 programs award a master's degree. Of those, several offer a choice of a certificate or master's degree, and one program awards a master's degree in public health (Whitfill & Burst, 1994). If faculty are planning curricula for CNM programs, given the trend, a master's program seems to be a wise choice. One interesting fact about the roles midwives perform is that in addition to their patient care functions, many participate in medical education (Harman, Summers, King, & Harman, 1998). One wonders if acceptance of advanced roles would increase if more advanced-practice nurses were involved collaboratively in medical education.

The number of CRNAs is approximately 21,800, and 6,017 have master's degrees (Health Resources and Services Administration, 1997).

Although the purpose of this review is not to evaluate fully the clinical outcomes observed of NPs and CNSs, brief mention should be made of recent studies that document the effectiveness of these roles because curricula should be designed to promote role performance. For example, Baradell (1994) found that as compared to psychologists, master's-prepared psychiatric clinical specialists delivered less costly care of equal quality. Ramsey, Edwards, Lenz, Odom, and Brown (1993) reported that 97% of a systematic sample of 101 clients surveyed via telephone were very satisfied with their care from family nurse practitioners, although the authors did not say whether master's-prepared clinicians delivered the care. Mahoney (1994) discovered that when nurse practitioners were compared to physicians on appropriateness of prescribing medications for the elderly, the NPs' practice was more appropriate even though the physicians had more years of experience. Again, no mention was made of the NPs' educational preparation.

Finally, Brown and Grimes (1995), conducting a meta-analysis of NPs and NMs employed in primary care, concluded that NPs and NMs provided care that was cost-effective and equal to or better than care provided by physicians. Their data did not speak to differences between master's-prepared and non-master's-prepared practitioners. However, one might assume that current curricula, including those at the master's level, are preparing graduates to meet the needs of patients in primary care settings.

Given the rapidly changing health care environment, many master's-prepared nurses might need further education to better function in the current advanced nursing practice roles. Therefore, nursing faculty might consider developing clinical programs at the postmaster's level. A survey published in the *Journal of the American Academy of Nurse Practitioners* ("What's Happening," 1994) supports this notion.

The aforementioned studies dealt exclusively with master's or postmaster's specialty educational preparation and their outcomes. One study, however, did explore specialty preparation at the doctoral level. Clarke et al. (1996) surveyed doctoral programs to determine the extent to which community health content was presented. Only four programs offered a major in community health, whereas the other 19 programs in the sample provided more general theoretical and research focused education. While this study only concentrated on community health, their findings support the fact that specialty preparation is almost exclusively within the purview of master's programs.

EDUCATOR AND RESEARCHER ROLES

The National League for Nursing (NLN, August 27, 1998) estimates that less than two-thirds of all nursing faculty have the master's degree as their highest credential; most of the remaining have doctoral degrees (see Table 7–1). A few faculty still have only the baccalaureate as the highest degree; perhaps these are located in practical nursing programs or serve as adjunct clinical faculty. Table 7–5 summarizes studies concerned with those who hold educator roles.

Since most master's programs have a heavy clinical emphasis, how faculty acquire skills for teaching is of some concern. Oermann and Jamison (1989) investigated the extent to which nursing education content was found in master's programs. The data showed that only 10 programs offered a major in nursing education, 34 programs offered minors, 18 programs had electives in nursing education, and 14 had tracks or other curricular designs. Fifteen programs had no nursing education courses. Numbers of credit hours in nursing education ranged from 2 to 20.

Because Canadians have a goal that professional nurses hold the baccalaureate degree for entry into practice by the year 2000, an adequate pool of faculty will be needed. Therefore, Ford and Wertenberger (1993) partially replicated, within the Canadian environment, Oermann and Jamison's study. One strength of their research report was that they included sample questions

TABLE 7–5.
Educator and Researcher Roles

Author/Date	Sample	Method	Findings
Clarke et al. (1996)	23 doctoral program directors, 16 faculty.	Mailed questionnaire, telephone interview.	Only four programs had community specialty in curriculum.
Farren (1991)	National sample of 152 doctorally prepared nurses.	Investigator-designed descriptive-correlational survey.	Employer support, type of degree, and participation in faculty research while a student correlated with current productivity.
Ford & Wertenberger (1993)	10 Canadian master's programs.	Survey using previously published instrument.	7 of 10 programs have nursing education coursework; 2 others require courses outside department.
Germain et al. (1994)	56 students, 22 alumni, 29 faculty.	ETS survey instruments.	Reported self-study process only.
Herrmann (1997)	692 faculty.	Investigator-designed and adapted questionnaire.	Little difference in teaching methods used between those who had teaching content in graduate program and those who did not.
Holzemer (1987)	14 doctoral programs.	Investigator-designed survey modified from previously published instruments.	Between 1979 and 1984, percentage of time faculty devoted to research increased.
Holzemer & Chambers (1986)	326 faculty, 659 students, 296 alumni.	Investigator-designed survey modified from previously published instruments.	Extramural funding was predictive of alumni productivity.
Hudacek & Carpenter (1998)	401 doctoral students.	Investigator-designed instrument based on previous study.	DNS students felt less prepared for quantitative research. Personal and professional growth same for all students.
Karuhije (1986)	211 nurse educators.	Investigator-designed survey.	Educators felt ill-prepared for clinical teaching role.
Keck (1992)	133 traditional MS students, 152 ITV students.	Quasi-experimental with intact groups.	Little difference in learning outcomes.
Ketefian & Lenz (1995)	38 doctoral programs.	Investigator-designed open-ended questionnaire.	Publication and authorship credit problematic. Standards for publication described.

TABLE 7–5.
Educator and Researcher Roles (Continued)

Author/Date	Sample	Method	Findings
Lash (1987)	31 doctoral programs.	Perusal of NLN documents.	Curricula differed little among various program types.
Lash (1992)	255 nurse doctorates from national sample.	Investigator-designed survey used for path analysis.	Graduation from top-ranked school an important predictor of career attainment.
Lott et al. (1993)	11 master's-prepared undergraduate faculty members.	Interviews analyzed thorough content analysis.	Faculty exhibit a variety of feelings and symptoms related to role stress and strain.
Megel et al. (1988)	148 leading nurse researchers.	Investigator-designed survey.	High producers identified with peers outside institution and taught less than low producers.
Oddi et al. (1994)	82 student authors who had published in *Image*.	Author-adapted previously used questionnaire.	Most publications resulted from dissertation work, but 13 from other coursework.
Oermann & Jamison (1989)	92 master's programs.	Investigator-designed survey.	10 programs offered nursing education major. Others had minors, electives, or tracks.
Olson & Connelly (1995)	4 student/faculty pairs.	Descriptive, qualitative.	Described value of mentoring process during predoctoral fellowship.
Reilly (1990)	One master's program.	Case study.	Outreach programs are a viable alternative for master's degree programs.
Sakalys et al. (1995)	76 doctoral students.	ETS questionnaire survey.	Summers-only prepared for teaching positions.
Snyder-Halpern (1986)	8 doctoral programs.	Case study.	PhD and DNSc programs were more alike than different.
Zebelman & Olswang (1989)	788 doctoral students from national sample.	Investigator-designed survey.	After first year of study, more students interested in research than teaching.

DNS = doctorate of nursing science
DNSc = doctorate of nursing science
ETC = Educational Testing Service

ITV = Interactive Television
MS = master of science
NLN = National League for Nursing

from the survey in a table. All 10 Canadian master's programs took part in their study. Results showed that dual role preparation was the norm and seven programs offered nursing education courses. Most programs offered one to two nursing education courses. While the purpose of the courses was to prepare nurse educators, coursework appeared to contain just an overview of knowledge and skills required for the teaching role. The authors suggested that more education coursework be required, but it could be offered in departments outside nursing. Since most nursing faculty in the United States are prepared at the master's level, curriculum planners may want to consider Ford and Wertenberger's suggested approach to providing additional coursework for potential nurse educators. Combining educational content taught within and outside a college of nursing might be the most efficacious way to teach students about educating students within higher education settings.

Investigating coursework required does shed some light on the extensiveness of preparation for the teaching role. However, faculty's perception of the adequacy of their preparation may help curriculum planners consider what might be needed in any curriculum revision. Karuhije (1986) used a convenience sample of educators who had attended an ADN workshop and faculty who attended an NLN convention. Data collection was via a very simple questionnaire, which was shown within the article. 78% of survey respondents agreed that their preparation for clinical teaching was inadequate. Essential content identified included clinical teaching strategies and clinical evaluation. Since few graduate programs emphasize the nurse educator role, faculty may want to integrate the identified essential content into a variety of course offerings.

Perceived adequacy of preparation is not the only issue; use of knowledge acquired is another element of whether an educational program produces desired outcomes. Herrmann (1997) discovered few relationships between formal coursework in educational theory and strategies and faculty's conduct of clinical courses. However, she noted that many in her sample were experienced educators who may have added to their repertoire of strategies through experience as a teacher.

Many facets of a master's-prepared educator's role can cause stress. Lott, Anderson, and Kenner (1993) used qualitative methods to examine how master's-prepared educators who teach in undergraduate programs in universities with doctoral programs cope with their environment. A thorough explanation of the study's methodology and data analysis showed that role theory formed the basis of the open-ended questions used in the interviews. Data disclosed that faculty felt like second-class citizens and perceived pressure to obtain a doctorate. Faculty viewed workload as inequitable among the undergraduate faculty but not between graduate and undergraduate faculty. Faculty recognized a variety of symptoms associated with stress, and to cope with this stress, faculty recommended more open communication between undergraduate and graduate faculty. They also wanted recognition for the contribution master's-prepared faculty make to the college's mission. To reduce role strain, the authors recommended that colleges help faculty achieve the doctoral degree by reducing workloads and encouraging faculty to develop buddy systems to cope with stress. The findings of Lott et al. would probably be supported by many other faculty employed in schools that have the full range of undergraduate and graduate curricula.

However, one wonders if faculty at universities without doctoral programs face the same stressors. To help faculty cope with stressors, perhaps teaching practicums should emphasize the totality of the faculty role, not just the actual teaching component. As a consequence, master's graduates might have a more realistic expectation of this role.

Ketefian (1991) and Fitzpatrick (1991) echoed similar sentiments by calling for doctoral programs to prepare students for all dimensions of the faculty role, even though the research role is stressed in doctoral programs. Nursing doctoral programs award primarily the PhD degree. Whether doctorate of nursing science (DNS or DNSc) programs differ substantially in their content devoted to preparing nurse researchers seems to have been clarified recently. Lash (1987) and Snyder-Halpern (1986) noted little difference, but Hudacek and Carpenter (1998) discovered that students in DNS programs felt preparation for quantitative research was less than in PhD programs, as was faculty mentorship for research. Doctorate of education (EdD) and DNS students felt better prepared for educator and clinician roles than did PhD students. Dennis (1991) stated that students need exposure to a variety of coursework and experiences that will foster research careers. Ketefian (1993) made a strong case for not only methodological courses but courses supported by substantive knowledge used to answer questions of interest to the discipline of nursing. Zebelman and Olswang (1989) found, from a nationwide survey of students in 35 doctoral programs, that the environment of the doctoral program encourages development of a career in research. After one year of study, students appeared to place greater value on developing research expertise than on other areas essential to faculty role performance. The authors commented that the desire for a research career may conflict with the actual demands of the environments where most would be employed.

Scholarly productivity is an expectation of graduates and employing institutions, particularly those with graduate programs. Lia-Hoagberg (1985) compared nursing faculty with doctorates to women in other academic fields employed at eight universities. More nonnurse faculty had research-focused careers, and nonnurse faculty had more publications. Nursing faculty had more administrative functions. One reason for this may have been that these nursing faculty were older and had not had the opportunity to develop their research foci.

Holzemer (1987) found that scholarly productivity of faculty increased from 1979 to 1984 as evidenced by the mean number of publications per faculty. The mean was 6.6 in 1979 and 7.4 in 1984. Although the difference was statistically nonsignificant, faculty devoted a greater percentage of time to research in 1984 at the $p = .01$ level. The number of dissertations supported by extramural funding was somewhat predictive of alumni productivity (Holzemer & Chambers, 1986).

Megel, Langston, and Creswell (1988) surveyed researchers who had been identified as top producers by deans at Research I and II universities and health science centers. Generally, high producers identified more with peers outside their institutions and their research team members. They also desired to conduct research more than to teach when compared to low producers. High producers continued to publish with graduate faculty advisors more than did low producers. One interesting finding, however, was that high producers spent more time on administrative duties than their low-producing peers. A strength of this study was the well-outlined methodology. A shortcoming was that the researchers did not use portions of Holzemer's instrumentation, nor was his work referenced.

Farren (1991) also examined faculty scholarly productivity, which was defined as the number of research projects (not the number of publications). Like Megel et al., she designed her own survey instrument without reference to previously published tools. She used a stratified random sample to gather data from nurses with various doctorates who were listed in the 1984 American Nurses Association Directory of Nurses with Doctoral Degrees. Individuals with doctorates other than nursing had a higher response rate (90%) than those with doctorates in nursing, whose response rate was 67.5%. Consistent with previous research, approximately two-thirds were employed in educational institutions. Seventy percent had conducted postdissertation research, which was a marked increase from other research cited by Farren. Computer experience and participating with faculty in research during their doctoral program were significantly correlated with current productivity. Nurses with PhDs and DNSs were more productive than those who held the EdD. Institutional support, such as released time and undefined employer support, also correlated with productivity. Similar to Megel et al.'s (1988) findings, Farren found that support from peers outside the employing institution was critical to productivity. Another interesting finding was that 42.8% felt able to conduct independent research, while 53.3% said they needed some assistance but were able to find that help.

Lash (1992) investigated variables related to the career attainment of faculty with doctoral degrees in nursing. She used the 1984 ANA directory and lists from the degree-granting institutions to identify this sample. A path analysis that described career variables in three stages—predoctorate, first job attainment, and current job attainment—was founded on prior research. A significant finding was that graduation from a top-ranked school predicted employment in a like institution. Numbers of publications were positively correlated with the ranking of the current employing institution, current faculty rank, and predoctoral teaching experience but not with predoctoral publications. Another finding of import was that faculty rank for the first job postgraduation was higher for those employed at lower ranked schools. The lower professorial rank persisted for those employed at higher ranked institutions, perhaps reflecting the more competitive environments in those schools. Lash stated that recognition by peers in the form of membership in honoraries and other like activities was also as a measure of career attainment. Predoctoral recognition and current publications contributed strongly to the recognition. Lash cautioned that expanding the numbers of doctoral programs might not be accompanied by an expansion of the quality and quantity of scholarly productivity for nursing as a whole.

Olson and Connelly (1995) confirmed that predoctoral experiences do enhance productivity. Using a case study approach they interviewed four student–faculty pairs. Results showed that the mentoring process that occurs in predoctoral fellowships is reciprocal between mentor and protégé, and the protégé was able to benefit from the socialization that supported the researcher role.

Graduate students also contribute to the body of nursing knowledge through paper presentation and publication (Oddi, Whitley, & Pool, 1994). Most articles were a result of dissertation work, but 13 articles (17%) in a sample identified as articles from student authors came from other coursework. Ketefian and Lenz (1995) stated that norms of scientific integrity require that if faculty publish with students, students should be first author on articles resulting from coursework or the dissertation.

Program evaluation is another avenue that may reveal how well those with doctorates are prepared for their various roles. Two studies were useful in this regard (Germain, Deatrick, Hagopian, & Whitney, 1994; Sakalys, Coates, & Chinn, 1995). Of note, both used standardized instruments from the Educational Testing Service (ETS) as part of the evaluation process. Since the evaluation process had not been completed at the time of their article's publication, Germain et al. (1994) only outlined their data collection plan. The plan involved data collection from various constituencies including alumni, faculty, and students. The details of the plan presented are sufficient enough for other doctoral programs to follow. Sakalys et al. (1995) did present the results of their evaluation of a summers-only doctoral program. Although the program was stressful, this scheduling option provided access to programs for students who might not otherwise have undertaken doctoral study. One important finding was that in comparison to regular academic-year students, summers-only students were preparing exclusively for teaching positions. The academic-year students were preparing for teaching/research or administration/management positions.

The fact that most doctoral program graduates will be employed in positions that involve at least some teaching further supports the idea that all components of the faculty role need emphasis in doctoral programs. Even though many doctoral candidates may already be experienced in teaching and service roles, they may need assurance that these roles will not be deemphasized if the research role is added.

NURSING ADMINISTRATORS

An estimated 28,500 nursing administrators hold master's degrees and approximately 3,400 have doctorates. The percentage of these degrees that are in nursing is unknown (Health Resources and Human Services Administration, 1997). Determining what knowledge and skills these administrators need seems particularly important if graduates are to serve as leaders in a turbulent health care system. However, the number of articles in the literature that could be used in curriculum planning was much lower than the number available for the clinical and educator roles (see Table 7–6).

Price (1984) surveyed graduates from master's programs with a major or functional component in nursing administration and their employers. A nursing administration program evaluation instrument was modified for use in her study. Over 50% of graduates expressed satisfaction with their education. Graduates from programs with solely an administrative focus thought their education contributed more to the effectiveness of their leadership skills than did graduates from other programs. No relationship existed between the level of graduates' perceived attainment of program goals and employer satisfaction with the graduates' performance. Graduates wanted more content in the area of financial management and, for the most part, did not perceive the need for advanced clinical knowledge.

Wagner, Henry, Giovinco, and Blanks (1988) analyzed 37 publications from the years 1976 to 1985 for recommendations regarding content for master's programs in nursing administration. They thoroughly described the content analysis and inter-rater reliability procedures. Data showed that content fell into the domains of organizational systems, political environment, economic concerns, and accounting and cost procedures. In addition, human resource management and work redesign seemed important. Twenty articles mentioned nursing theoretical foundations, but only two referred to clinical specialization. These findings seem to support content identified as relevant by the respondents in Price's (1984) study.

Minnick (1993) contacted students enrolled in MSN programs, dual MBA/MSN programs, and a variety of other dual-degree programs. She chose the single-focus programs sampled according to similar geographic distribution and academic ratings as compared to the dual-degree programs. Several findings of note emerged. Dual-degree students were more likely to study full time and seek employment outside a hospital setting. Some of these students stated that they would have attended MBA programs only if a dual-degree program had not been available. The author postulated that the brightest students may be attracted to these dual-degree programs, because their scores on the GRE were higher than MSN students. In other words, these bright students might have been lost to nursing if the dual-degree program had not been available. Given this finding, nursing graduate faculties might want to incorporate more administrative content into their programs in order to attract these bright students.

The previous studies concentrated, for the most part, on student and graduate perceptions of needed content and skills. Smith (1993), however, explored important skills for effective management from the perspective of the manager. Using a theoretical model derived from Katz (1974), Smith constructed a reliable and valid survey tool, which she sent to a stratified random sample of directors of nursing (presumably the chief nurse executive) at member hospitals of the College of Teaching Hospitals. She placed questionnaire items, shown within tables

TABLE 7–6.
Nurse Administrators

Author/Date	Sample	Method	Findings
Haynor & Wells (1998)	48 graduate nursing administration programs.	Previously used questionnaire.	Enrollments declining in major. Recommends program redesign.
Parsons et al. (1998)	40 nurse executives, 56 persons who had influenced careers.	Investigator-designed survey.	Graduate degree necessary for effective role performance. Importance of mentor or role model for career progression.
Minnick (1993)	279 MSN students, 57 MSN/MBA dual-degree students, 23 other students.	Investigator-designed survey.	Dual-degree students more likely to seek jobs outside hospital. Dual-degree programs may keep students within nursing.
Price (1984)	10 nursing administration master's programs.	Survey using previously published instrument.	Described overview of curricula.
Smith (1993)	75 directors of nursing.	Investigator-designed survey.	Needed skills included conceptual, human, and technical.
Wagner et al. (1988)	37 publications.	Content analysis.	Important content areas included health policy, nursing practice, research, and finance.

MBA = master of business administration
MSN = master of science–nursing

in the article, into the categories of conceptual, human, and technical skills. Directors acknowledged the importance of conceptual skills such as analyzing the political dimensions of the work environment and designing and implementing organizational structure, but they saw a need for improved performance in these areas. Directors said human skills such as interpersonal communication needed improvement, and they rated skills in this domain as highly important for effective performance. Only 18.3% of the directors reported conflicting expectations of the educational program and job requirements with regard to technical skills such as financial management. For all skill dimensions, a positive correlation existed between self-assessment and importance of skill behaviors. These skill dimensions were similar in nature to those identified by Price (1984) and Wagner et al. (1988).

Parsons, Fosbinder, Murray, and Dwore (1998) noted that 78% of their sample of 48 nurse executives felt that a graduate degree was essential for their job performance, but the need for formal education ranked second to having a mentor. The nurse executives and their mentors also stated that better preparation was needed to deal with systems issues. Areas of additional preparation included information technology, strategic planning, financial management, and systems management including physician–hospital organizations.

One trend evidenced in the studies concerned with the nursing administrator role is that many of the skills are of an interdisciplinary nature and do not involve advanced clinical skills. Because administrators have to work within an interdisciplinary environment daily, faculty must consider locating some coursework for potential administrators in an interdisciplinary environment and strengthening skills needed to deal with complex systems issues.

The health care delivery system has changed rapidly in last decade, and the need for adequately prepared nursing administrators is more acute than ever before. Yet the number of programs in nursing administration has decreased (Haynor and Wells, 1998). Some have even questioned whether nursing administrators should be prepared in nursing programs at all (Malloch, 1998). However, as Haynor and Wells point out, a drastic revision in nursing administration curricula will allow nursing administrators to maintain their clinical leadership and at the same time be proficient in today's business-oriented health care environment.

INTERNATIONAL GRADUATE EDUCATION OUTCOMES

Adequate preparation for advanced practice roles is of concern to those outside the United States as well (see Table 7–7). Needs assessments in Hong Kong, Northern Ireland, and England have shown the necessity of graduate preparation for advanced-practice roles. A survey of nurses in Hong Kong showed that 50% of 705 survey participants desired specialist education at the master's level (Simsen, Holroyd, & Sellick, 1996). To provide for a variety of advanced-practice nurses, the University of Ulster designed a program that allowed

TABLE 7-7.
The State and Outcomes of International Graduate Education

Author/Date	Sample	Method	Findings
Alcock (1996)	208 Ontario health care agencies.	Investigator-designed survey.	Community health centers and academic health centers employ most CNSs and NPs. Multiplicity of other titled nurses.
Boore (1996)	One university.	Case study.	Description of graduate program with multiple exits.
Duffield et al. (1995)	373 Australian CNSs.	Survey adapted from previously used questionnaire.	CNSs not all master's prepared. Have more financial functions than CNSs in U.S.
McGee et al. (1996)	230 senior British Health Trust nurses.	Investigator-designed survey.	Little use of ANPs. Wide use of specialist nurses.
Pelletier et al. (1994)	40 Australian RNs enrolled in graduate study.	Longitudinal study.	Career advancement prime motivator for graduate study.
Simpson (1997)	39 Canadian postmaster's acute care nurse practitioners.	Longitudinal study.	Retained nursing expertise and 6 months after graduation variable skill with medical tasks.
Simsen et al. (1996)	705 Hong Kong nurses.	Investigator-designed survey.	Preference for specialist programs offered part time.

ANP = adult nurse practitioner
CNS = certified nurse specialist
NP = nurse practitioner
RN = registered nurse
APN = advanced practice nurse

nurses to exit with a postgraduate diploma in midwifery, an MS degree, or a DNSc (Boore, 1996). Before the program's inception, students had little opportunity for graduate education in nursing. Students in this part-time program noted that they benefitted from an advanced theoretical understanding of clinical problems and increased understanding of research.

Confusion over titles is also an issue in the international arena. Alcock (1996) examined titles of advanced-practice nurses in Ontario and found that most clinical nurse specialists and clinical nurse specialists/nurse practitioners were employed in teaching hospitals. Other titled nurses such as diabetic educators were employed primarily in community hospitals. While the functions of the nurse specialists and practitioners were in line with published literature, the other titled nurses had varying roles and functions. Further, the author questioned why nurses who have acquired specialty expertise are retitled, particularly if their scope of practice is not clearly delineated. The author also stated that the demand for clinical nurse specialists/nurse practitioners would increase in the next nine years.

Canadians also seem to have followed the trend in developing acute care nurse practitioner programs. Simpson (1997) reported the outcomes of a fast-track acute care nurse practitioner program. The three-month program enrolled master's-prepared nurses who were already functioning in an advanced-practice role. The students were employer sponsored. Six months following program completion, students met with an external consultant and reviewer. The consultant evaluated case studies to see if the students were functioning as expected. The outcomes of the case studies were used for further program development. Case studies showed that students were strong in their previously honed specialist functions but required further development in constructing treatment plans based on laboratory and other diagnostic information. Most had strong nursing knowledge and were working to integrate the medical component of their role. Physician and nurse employers were very satisfied with the graduates' performance; however, the author did not specifically address the impact of prior experience upon actual performance as an acute nurse practitioner.

Australians, too, are interested in the components of advanced practice roles, but because graduate education is relatively new in that country, those in advanced-practice roles may not always have graduate degrees. Duffield, Donoghue, and Pelletier (1995) conducted a study of 373 clinical nurse specialists. The nurses were specialists by virtue of their experience in a specialty area or experience and education beyond the basic program. As compared to specialists in the United States, Australian nurse specialists have more responsibilities in the financial arena. Role confusion emerged as the nurse specialists seemed to have overlapping functions with nurse managers; some of this confusion was attributed to the cost-conscious health care environment.

Pelletier et al. (1994) explored the effects of graduate education on career paths and practice patterns. They used an investigator-designed instrument to gather data about 22 graduates upon graduation, and they sought permission to collect longitudinal data. Most subjects furthered their education in order to advance their careers and increase their job opportunities. Students gained increased confidence, but 30% noted negative effects on personal health and stress levels.

Expectations of employers of advanced-practice nurses were the concern of McGee, Castledine, and Brown (1996), who surveyed 371 National Health Trusts in England to determine role expectations of those in advanced and specialist roles. Definitions of these roles were similar to definitions in the United States, but this particular article did not speak to the educational qualifications of nurses who fulfilled these roles. Findings showed that nurse specialists were more widely employed than advanced nurse practitioners. Functions of the specialists and the practitioners were in line with the role definitions. Respondents were concerned, however, with overspecialization of nurses and possible "de-skilling" of doctors and other nurses. Other findings included low pay rates and confusion between the specialist nurse and practitioner roles.

SUMMARY

A voluminous amount of research exists regarding the utilization of graduates from master's and doctoral programs. Since the first edition of this chapter, in addition to national data sets from the federal government and national surveys sponsored by professional organizations, states have published their own data regarding the utilization of advanced practice nurses. These data provide program planning support for university-specific curricula as well as university-specific follow-up of master's graduates.

Many studies of doctoral programs were national in scope, perhaps because the target population was smaller. Data were gathered primarily through investigator-designed instruments, and study conclusions were drawn mainly from descriptive correlational statistics. Lash's (1992) study was a notable exception; additionally, Sakalys et al. (1995) and Germain et al. (1994) used standardized instruments for data collection (vs. investigator-designed instruments). Studying utilization and effectiveness of nurses in advanced clinical practice, however, was amenable to other means, as evidenced by Fenton and Brykczynski's (1993) work.

Although many of the studies were limited in scope, a consensus of findings seemed to emerge. Graduates from master's programs and their employers want nurses who can function in multiple roles. Both clinical nurse specialists and nurse practitioners need to have a core of advanced nursing knowledge that will allow them to function in a variety of settings. The demand for clinical knowledge has remained stable over time, but acquisition of such knowledge is not sufficient for effective role performance. Most advanced nurse practitioners need some administrative skills and knowledge to function competently in the complex organizations in which they work. Administrators, on the other hand, may need more knowledge and skills in the administrative arena and less in the clinical, while at the same time maintaining a deep understanding of the realities and requirements of clinical settings.

Most doctoral program graduates work in academic institutions that place multiple demands on their time. Many graduates expect that research will be a priority in their careers; however, with the exception of those in top-ranked Research I universities, teaching may take a higher priority. For educators with a master's degree, role confusion and stress will continue as they try to compete with doctorally prepared faculty for resources to support their careers.

Finally, the international climate seems similar to that in the United States with regard to role performance of graduates. However, the need for more graduate programs was evidenced by the fact that more nurses outside the United States, as compared to within the United States, may be functioning in advanced roles without graduate degrees.

CONCLUSIONS

Anticipating how nursing curricula should be changed to prepare graduates for an ever-changing health care system is challenging, to say the least. A Report to Congress (Health Resources and Services Administration, 1990) states that the need for those with master's and doctoral degrees will grow. The more recent Pew Commission (1995) and Institute of Medicine (1996) reports echo this appraisal. While the total of employed nurses with master's degrees is estimated to be 193,159, the projected demand is for 363,000 (Health Resources and Services Administration, 1990, 1997). Recent data confirm that an increased demand for health services along with an aging nursing workforce places challenges on meeting this demand (Buerhaus, 1998). Not only must the numbers of graduates increase, but educators will have to find innovative ways to educate students who can be flexible in meeting the needs of the health care system. One report suggests that an argument against required master's preparation for nurse practitioners is lack of available programs in rural and underserved areas (Fowkes, Gamel, Garcia, Wilson, & Stewart, 1993). Others argue that distance learning strategies could be used for students in these geographical areas without compromising quality (Keck, 1992; Reilly, 1990; Tagg & Arreola, 1996).

Changing demographics will necessitate curricula that address the needs of the elderly in primary and long-term care settings. Health care system complexity will also require that graduates have excellent communication skills in order to function effectively in interdisciplinary environments (Lenz, 1994).

As the need for master's graduates increases, a concomitant need for doctorally prepared faculty will increase. Full-time faculty line vacancies have increased slightly in the past several years (NLN, personal communication, August 27, 1998). The increased use of part-time faculty and perhaps the lack of qualified full-time faculty have caused some universities to recapture the nursing lines and reallocate them to other departments. However, as current faculty retire, the need for faculty may further outweigh the supply. Therefore, doctoral program faculty will have to find ways to educate students who cannot attend school full-time, perhaps through outreach, weekend, and summer programs. In that environment, mentoring students in a way that fosters their academic careers will be challenging.

Both master's and doctoral administrators and faculty may want to rethink the current trend to deemphasize teaching role development. If those with advanced degrees are to work in academic environments, they should have formal preparation. This lack of preparation is not unique to the discipline of nursing. Nursing has had a strong heritage with regard to preparation for faculty roles, but this preparation has been lost as many master's-level programs have focused on advanced clinical practice and doctoral programs have emphasized preparation for research careers.

Providing master's and doctoral programs that use flexible teaching/learning strategies will not be enough. Nursing faculty must have a constant sense of what skills and knowledge are needed to function in an uncertain environment. To that end, local follow-up studies of graduates and their employers may give useful information; however, larger cross-institutional studies may better facilitate local, state, regional, and federal planning. Institutions could share data collection instruments rather than developing them independently, or institutions should be encouraged to use the standardized instruments that are available so data can be pooled and compared. Further, using standardized instruments to collect data could assist schools and accrediting agencies in defining and documenting achievement of required outcomes of academic programs. Studies using qualitative methodologies could help faculty better understand the nuances of advanced practice so they could better incorporate the realities of the practice environment into their educational programs.

The research suggests that the most productive doctorally prepared faculty, in terms of scholarship, are concentrated in the top-ranked schools, and given the available funding resources, this pattern is likely to continue. However, a need will continue to exist for doctoral education outside the top-ranked schools. Perhaps those schools should prepare students who can meet the demands of faculty roles in places that are not centers of research excellence but do provide top-quality undergraduate and graduate education. Those faculty whose primary emphasis is teaching might focus their scholarship on advanced clinical practice and the teaching/learning process, and they might conduct research in partnerships with the major universities. Talent exists nationwide, and multiinstitution collaboration will help capture that talent and advance the discipline of nursing.

Finally, with accrediting agencies focusing on documenting outcomes, there is a critical need for faculty to publish studies that describe the data collected vis-à-vis the outcomes. These studies need to present evidence for (or lack thereof) the validity and reliability of the measurement of those outcomes. While focusing on outcomes is a worthy effort, it is just as important to investigate whether or not the outcomes are relevant, have been precisely defined, and have been measured appropriately. These data need to be reported in a timely manner, because reporting data that are more than several years old often is not useful to the reader. Perhaps such data should be reported in peer-reviewed on-line journals that publish the data immediately following peer review, rather than the usual 1 or more years later as is common with printed journals.

Graduate programs have a vital role to play in providing education for advanced nurse practitioners, faculty, researchers, and administrators. Continued research on the utilization and effectiveness of graduates will help faculty improve current curricula and plan for the future health care system.

REFERENCES

Alcock, D. S. (1996). The clinical nurse specialist, clinical nurse specialist/ nurse practitioner and other titled nurse in Ontario. *Canadian Journal of Nursing Administration,* 9(1), 23–44.

American Association of Colleges of Nursing. (1996). The essentials of master's education for advanced practice nursing. Washington, DC: Author.

American Nurses Association. *Directory of nurses with doctoral degrees* (Publication No. G-143). Kansas City, MO: Author.

American Nurses Association. (1992). *Nursing's agenda for health care reform* (Publication No. PR-3). Washington, DC: Author.

Bachman, J. (1995). A university's response to a need for school nurse education. *Journal of School Nursing,* 11(3), 20–24.

Baradell, J. G. (1994). Cost-effectiveness and quality of care provided by clinical nurse specialists. *Journal of Psychosocial Nursing,* 32(3), 21–24.

Barkauskas, V. H., & Blaha, A. J. (1989). A survey of home care programs. *Caring,* 8(2), 16–20.

Beal, J. A., Maguire, D., & Carr, R.(1996). Neonatal nurse practitioners: Identity as advanced practice nurses. *Journal of Obstetrics, Gynecology, and Neonatal Nursing,* 25, 401–406.

Benner, P. (1984). *From novice to expert.* Menlo Park, CA: Addison-Wesley.

Boore, J. R. P. (1996). Postgraduate education in nursing: A case study. *Journal of Advanced Nursing,* 23, 620–629.

Brimmer, P. F., Skoner, M. M., Pender, N. J., Williams, C. A., Fleming, J. W., & Werley, H. H. (1983). Nurses with doctoral degrees: Education and employment characteristics. *Research in Nursing and Health,* 6, 157–165.

Brophy, E. B., Rankin, D., Butler, S., & Egenes, K. (1989). The master's prepared mental health nurse: An assessment of employer expectations. *Journal of Nursing Education,* 28, 156–160.

Brown, J. M. (1978). Master's education in nursing, 1945–1969. In M. Louise Fitzpatrick (Ed.), *Historical studies in nursing* (pp. 104–130). New York: Teachers College Press.

Brown, S. A., & Grimes, D. E. (1995). A meta-analysis of nurse practitioners and nurse midwives in primary care. *Nursing Research,* 44, 332–339.

Buchanan, L. (1996). The acute care nurse practitioner in collaborative practice. *Journal of the American Academy of Nurse Practitioners,* 8, 13–20.

Buerhaus, P. (1998, September). *Nurse labor market: New demands for quality and patient care.* Paper presented at the meeting of the Midwest Alliance in Nursing, Indianapolis, IN.

Burns, P. G., Nishikawa, H. A., Weatherby, F., Forni, P. R., Moran, M., & Allen, M. E. (1993). Master's degree nursing education: State of the art. *Journal of Professional Nursing, 9,* 267–277.

Busen, N. H., & Jones, M. E. (1995). Leadership development: Educating nurse practitioners for the future. *Journal of the American Academy of Nurse Practitioners, 7,* 111–117.

Cairo, M. J. (1996). Emergency physicians' attitudes toward the emergency nurse practitioner role: Validation versus rejection. *Journal of the American Academy of Nurse Practitioners, 8,* 411–417.

Caldwell, M. A., Wood, C. M., & Dibble, S. L. (1996). Cardiovascular clinical nurse specialists: Demographic, practice, and educational characteristics. *Progress in Cardiovascular Nursing, 11*(3), 23–32.

Cannon, J., & Beare, P. G. (1997). The utilization of master's prepared nurses in hospitals and parish health units in Louisiana. *Pelican News, 53*(5), 6–9. (Text from CINAHL on-line)

Chamberlin, E. M., & Rogers, B. (1997). Credentialing study: An AAOHN study. *AAOHN Journal, 45,* 431–437.

Chase, L. K., Johnson, S. K., Laffoon, T. A., Jacobs, R. S., & Johnson, M. E. (1996). CNS role: An experience in retitling and role clarification. *Clinical Nurse Specialist, 10,* 41–45.

Christensen, M., Richard, E., Froberg, D., McGovern, P., & Abanobi, O. C. (1985). An analysis of the employment patterns, roles, and functions of master's prepared occupational health nurses: Part II. *Occupational Health Nursing, 33,* 453–459.

Clarke, P. N., Glick, D. F., Laffrey, S. C., Bender, K., Emerson, S. E., & Stanhope, M. (1996). Doctoral education in community health nursing: A national survey. *Journal of Professional Nursing, 12,* 303–310.

Cronenwett, L. (1995). Molding the future for advanced practice nurses: Education, regulation, and practice. In *Role differentiation of the nurse practitioner and clinical nurse specialist: Reaching toward consensus* (pp. 1–20). Washington, DC: American Association of Colleges of Nursing.

Dennis, K. E. (1991). Components of the doctoral curriculum that build success in the clinical nurse researcher role. *Journal of Professional Education, 7,* 160–165.

Derstine, J. B. (1992). The rehabilitation clinical nurse specialist of the 1990s: Roles assumed by recent graduates. *Rehabilitation Nursing, 17,* 139–140.

Duffield, C., Donoghue, J., & Pelletier, D. (1995). CNSs' perceptions of role competencies: One Australian perspective. *Clinical Nurse Specialist, 9,* 13–22.

Dunn, A. M. (1993a). 1992 NAPNAP membership survey: Part I. Member characteristics, issues, and opinions. *Journal of Pediatric Health Care, 7,* 245–250.

Dunn, A. M. (1993b). 1992 NAPNAP membership survey: Part II. Practice characteristics of pediatric nurse practitioners indicate greater autonomy for PNPs. *Journal of Pediatric Health Care, 7,* 296–302.

Elder, R. G., & Bullough, B. (1990). Nurse practitioners and clinical specialists: Are the roles merging? *Clinical Nurse Specialist, 4,* 78–84.

Farren, E. A. (1991). Doctoral preparation and research productivity. *Nursing Outlook, 39,* 22–25.

Fenton, M. V. (1992). Education for the advanced practice of clinical nurse specialists. *Oncology Nursing Forum, 19* (Suppl. 1), 16–20.

Fenton, M. V., & Brykczynski, K. A. (1993). *Journal of Professional Nursing, 9,* 313–326.

Fitzpatrick, M. L. (1991). Doctoral preparation versus expectations. *Journal of Professional Nursing, 7,* 172–176.

Forbes, K. E., Rafson, J., Spross, J. A., & Kozlowski, D. (1990). Clinical nurse specialist and nurse practitioner core curricula survey results. *Nurse Practitioner, 17*(4), 43–48.

Ford, J. S., & Wertenberger, D. H. (1993). Nursing education content in master's in nursing programs. *Canadian Journal of Nursing Education, 25*(2), 53–61.

Fowkes, V., Gamel, N. N., Garcia, R. D., Wilson, S. R., & Stewart, B. R. (1993). *Assessment of physician assistant (PA), nurse practitioner (NP), and nurse-midwife (CNM) training on meeting health-care needs of the underserved* (Contract No. 240-91-0050). Rockville, MD: Office of Program Development, Bureau of Health Professions.

Frank, B. (1996). Utilization of master's and doctoral program graduates: Implications for curricula. In K. R. Stevens (Ed.), *Review of research in nursing education: Volume VII* (pp. 148–175). New York: National League for Nursing.

Frauman, A. C., & Germino, B. (1998). Survey of nephrology nurses' interest in graduate education. *ANNA Journal, 25*(1), 59–61.

Froerer, R. (1998). The nurse endoscopist: Reality or fiction? *Gastroenterology Nursing, 21*(1), 14–20.

Gallagher, J., Spross, J. A., & Powel, L. L. (1992). Introduction and overview of the conference. *Oncology Nursing Forum* (Suppl. 1), 7–10.

Germain, G. P., Deatrick, J. A., Hagopian, G. A., & Whitney, F. W. (1994). Evaluation of a PhD program: Paving the way. *Nursing Outlook, 41,* 117–122.

Gieske, M. (1995). Academic and demographic variables related to completion status of nursing students in master's degree programs. *Journal of Nursing Education, 34,* 282–285.

Guzik, V. L., McGovern, P. M., & Kochervar, L. K. (1992). Role function and job satisfaction. *AAOHN Journal, 40,* 521–530.

Hansen, M. J., & Pozehl, B. J. (1995). The effectiveness of admission criteria in predicting achievement in a master's degree program in nursing. *Journal of Nursing Education, 34,* 433–436.

Harman, P.J., Summers, L., King, T., & Harman, T. F. (1998). Collaborative practice issues: medical education: interdisciplinary teaching: a survey of CNM participation in medical education in the United States. *Journal of Nurse-Midwifery, 43,* 1, pp. 27–37.

Haw, M. A. (1996). Case management education in universities: A national survey. *The Journal of Care Management, 2*(6), 10–23.

Haynor, P. H., & Wells, R. W. (1998). Will nursing administration programs survive in the 21st century? *Journal of Nursing Administration, 28*(1), 15–24.

Health Resources and Services Administration. (1990). *Report to Congress on the study of need for nurse advanced trained specialists* (NTIS No. PB 91-105155). Rockville, MD: author.

Health Resources and Services Administration. (1994a). The registered nurse population: *Findings from the national sample survey of registered nurses, March 1992* (ISBN 0-16-042616-2). Washington, DC: U.S. Government Printing Office.

Health Resources and Services Administration. (1994b). *Survey of certified nurse practitioners and clinical nurse specialists: December 1992* (NTIS No. PB 94-158169). Rockville, MD: author.

Health Resources and Services Administration. (1997). *The registered nurse population: Findings from the national survey of registered nurses, March 1996*. Rockville, MD: Department of Health and Human Services, Bureau of Health Professions.

Heller, B. R., Damrosch, S. P., Romano, C. A., & McCarthy, M. R. (1989). Graduate specialization in nursing informatics. *Computers in Nursing, 7*, 68–76.

Herrmann, M. M. (1997). The relationship between graduate preparation and clinical teaching in nursing. *Journal of Nursing Education, 36*, 317–322.

Hill, B. A. (1989). The development of a master's degree program based on perceived future needs. *Journal of Nursing Education, 28*, 307–313.

Holzemer, W. L. (1987). Doctoral education in nursing: An assessment in quality, 1979–1984. *Nursing Research, 36*, 111–116.

Holzemer, W. L., & Chambers, D. B. (1986). Healthy doctoral programs: Relationship between perceptions of the academic environment and productivity of faculty and alumni. *Research in Nursing and Health, 9*, 299–307.

Hudacek, S., & Carpenter, D. M. (1994). Doctoral education in nursing: A comprehensive review of the research and theoretical literature. In L. R. Allen (Ed.), *Review of research in nursing education: Vol VI* (pp. 57–90). New York: National League for Nursing.

Hudacek, S., & Carpenter, D. M. (1998). Student perceptions of nurse doctorates: Similarities and differences. *Journal of Professional Nursing, 14*, 14–21.

Hungler, B. P., Krawczyk, R., Joyce, A., & Polit, D. (1979). Professionalism in nursing master's graduates. *Journal of Advanced Nursing, 4*, 193–203.

Ingersoll, G. L. (1995). Evaluation of the advanced practice nurse role in acute and specialty care. *Critical Care Nursing Clinics of North America, 7*(1), 25–33.

Jacobs, M., Wyman, J. F., Rowell, P., & Smith, D. A. (1998). Continence nurses: A survey of who they are and what they do. *Urological Nursing, 18*(1), 13–20.

Johnson, P. (1996). Nursing demographics and the provision of primary care in North Carolina: Presentation before the Health Care Reform Commission January 24, 1996. *Tar Heel Nurse, 58*(2), 10–12. (Text from CINAHL on-line)

Katz, R. L. (1974). Skills of an effective administrator. *Harvard Business Review, 52,* 90–102.

Karuhije, H. F. (1986). Educational preparation for clinical teaching: Perceptions of nurse educators. *Journal of Nursing Education, 25,* 137–144.

Keck, J. F. (1992). Comparison of learning outcomes between graduate students in telecourses and those in traditional classrooms. *Journal of Nursing Education, 31,* 229–234.

Ketefian, S. (1991). Doctoral preparation for faculty roles: Expectations and realities. *Journal of Professional Nursing, 7,* 105–111.

Ketefian, S. (1993). Essentials of doctoral education: Organization of program around knowledge areas. *Journal of Professional Nursing, 9,* 255–261.

Ketefian, S., & Lenz, E. R. (1995). Promoting integrity in nursing research: Part II. Strategies. *Journal of Professional Nursing, 11,* 263–269.

Kinney, A. Y., Hawkins, R., & Hudman, K. S. (1997). A descriptive study of the role of the oncology nurse practitioner. *Oncology Nursing Forum, 24,* 811–820.

Kleinpell, R. M. (1997). Acute-care nurse practitioners: Roles and practice profiles. *AACN Clinical Issues, 8*(1), 156–162.

Lash, A. A. (1987). Rival conceptions in doctoral education in nursing and their outcomes: An update. *Journal of Nursing Education, 26,* 221–227.

Lash, A. A. (1992). Determinants of career attainments of doctorates in nursing. *Nursing Research, 41,* 216–222.

Lenz, E. R. (1994). Paradigm shifts, changing contexts, and graduate nursing education. Paper presented at a regional meeting of the Southern Council on Collegiate Education for Nursing (SNRS). In SNRS, *A changing health care system: How will it affect advanced nursing education and practice?* Atlanta: Southern Council on Collegiate Education in Nursing, pp. 19–22.

Lia-Hoagberg, B. (1985). Comparison of professional activities of nurse doctorates and other academic women. *Nursing Research, 34,* 155–159.

Lindeke, L. L., Canedy, B. H., & Kay, M. M. (1997). A comparison of practice domains of clinical nurse specialists and nurse practitioners. *Journal of Professional Nursing, 13,* 281–287.

Lott, J. W., Anderson, E. R., & Kenner, C. (1993). Role stress and strain among nondoctorally prepared undergraduate faculty in a school of nursing with a doctoral program. *Journal of Professional Nursing, 9,* 14–22.

Louis, M., & Sabo, C. E. (1994). Nurse practitioners: Need for and willingness to hire as viewed by nurse administrators, nurse practitioners, and physicians. *Journal of the American Academy of Nurse Practitioners, 6,* 113–119.

Mahoney, D. F. (1994). The appropriateness of geriatric prescribing decisions made by nurse practitioners and physicians. *Image: The Journal of Nursing Scholarship, 26,* 41–46.

Malloch, K. (1998). In my opinion: The demise of nursing administration graduate programs. *Journal of Nursing Administration, 28*(7/8), 14–15.

McGee, P., Castledine, G., & Brown, R. (1996). A survey of specialist and advanced practice nursing in England. *British Journal of Nursing, 5,* 682–686.

McGovern, P., Richard, E., Christensen, M., Froberg, D., & Abanobi, O. C. (1985). An analysis of the employment patterns, roles and functions of master's prepared occupational health nurses: Part I. *Occupational Health Nursing, 33,* 407–413.

McLane, A. M. (1978). Core competencies of master's-prepared nurses. *Nursing Research, 27,* 48–53.

Megel, M. E., Langston, N. F., & Creswell, J. W. (1988). Scholarly productivity: A survey of nursing faculty researchers. *Journal of Professional Nursing, 4,* 45–54.

Melkus, G. D., & Fain, J. (1995). Diabetes care concentration: A program of study for advanced practice nurses. *Clinical Nurse Specialist, 9,* 313–316.

Minnick, A. (1993). MSN in nursing administration and the dual degree. *Nursing and Health Care, 14,* 22–26.

Oddi, L. F., Whitley, G. G., & Pool, B. J. (1994). Contributions of graduate students to the creation and dissemination of nursing knowledge. *Image: Journal of Nursing Scholarship, 26,* 7–11.

Oermann, M. H., & Jamison, M. T. (1989). Nursing education component in master's programs. *Journal of Nursing Education, 28,* 252–255.

Olson, R. K. & Connelly, L. M. (1995). Mentoring through predoctoral fellowships to enhance research productivity. *Journal of Professional Nursing, 11,* 270–275.

O'Sullivan, P. S., Blevins-Stephens, W. L., Smith, F. M., & Vaughn-Wrobel, B. (1997). Addressing the National League for Nursing critical-thinking outcome. *Nurse Educator, 22*(1), 23–29.

Parsons, R. J., Fosbinder, D., Murray, B., & Dwore, R. B. (1998). Spotlight on: Attributes of successful nurse executives: Survey of nurses and their mentors. *Journal of Nursing Administration, 28*(7/8), 10–13.

Pelletier, D., Duffield, C., Gallagher, R., Soars, L., Donoghue, J., & Adams, A. (1994). The effects of graduate nurse education on clinical practice and career paths: A pilot study. *Nurse Education Today, 14,* 314–321.

Pew Health Professions Commission. (1995). *Critical challenge: Revitalizing the health professions for the twenty-first century.* San Francisco: Pew Health Professions.

Pitts, J., & Seimer, B. (1998). The use of nurse practitioners in pediatric institutions. *Journal of Pediatric Health Care, 12*(2), 67–72.

Price, S. A. (1984). Master's programs preparing nursing administrators: What are the essential components? *Journal of Nursing Administration, 14*(1), 11–17.

Radke, K., McArt, E., Schmitt, M., & Walker, E. K. (1990). Administrative preparation of clinical nurse specialists. *Journal of Professional Nursing, 6,* 221–228.

Ramsey, P., Edwards, J., Lenz, C., Odom, J. E., & Brown, B. (1993). Types of health problems and satisfaction with services in a rural nurse-managed clinic. *Journal of Community Health Nursing, 10,* 161–170.

Reilly, D. E. (1990). *Graduate professional education through outreach: A nursing case study.* New York: National League for Nursing.

Ryan, M., & Carlton, K. H. (1997). Portfolio applications in a school of nursing. *Nurse Educator, 22*(1), 35–39.

Ruth-Sanchez, V., Lee, K. A., & Bosque, E. M. (1996). A descriptive study of current neonatal nurse practitioner practice. *Neonatal Network, 15*(5), 23–29.

Sakalys, J. A., Coates, C. J., & Chinn, P. L. (1995). Doctoral education in nursing: Evaluation of a nontraditional program option. *Journal of Professional Nursing, 11,* 281–289.

Segall, M., & McKay, R. (1984). Evolution of an aggregate-based community health curriculum. *Nursing Outlook, 32,* 308–312.

Selby, M. L., Riportella-Muller, R., Salmon, M. E., Legault, C., & Quade, D. (1991). Master's degree-level community health nursing educational needs: A national survey of leaders on service and education. *Journal of Professional Nursing, 7,* 88–98.

Simpson, B. (1997). An educational partnership to develop acute care nurse practitioners. *Canadian Journal of Nursing Administration, 10*(1), 69–84.

Simsen, B. J., Holyroyd, E., & Sellick, K. (1996). Postgraduate education expectations: A survey of Hong Kong graduate nurses. *Journal of Advanced Nursing, 24,* 827–835.

Smith, M. C. (1980). Evaluation of master's program by graduates and their employers. *Journal of Nursing Education, 19*(9), 4–10.

Smith, P., Moody, N., Glenn, L. L., & Garmany, J. D. (1996). Nurse practitioner research network: Patterns of practice in northeast Tennessee. *Tennessee Nurse, 59*(2), 25–26. (Text from CINAHL on-line)

Smith, T. (1993). Management skills for directors of nursing. *Journal of Nursing Administration, 23*(9), 38–49.

Snyder-Halpern, R. (1986). Doctoral programs in nursing: An examination of curriculum similarities and differences. *Journal of Nursing Education, 25,* 359–365.

Stokes, E., Whitis, G., & Moore-Thrasher, L. (1997). Characteristics of graduate adult health nursing programs. *Journal of Nursing Education, 36,* 54–59.

Tagg, P. I., & Arreola, R. A. (1996). Earning a master's of science in nursing degree in nursing through distance education. *Journal of Professional Nursing, 12,* 154–158.

Towers, J. (1989). Part I: Report of the American Academy of Nurse Practitioners national nurse practitioner survey. *Journal of the American Academy of Nurse Practitioners, 1,* 91–94.

Towers, J. (1990). Report of the national survey of the American Academy of Nurse Practitioners, Part IV: Practice characteristics and marketing activities of nurse practitioners. *Journal of the American Academy of Nurse Practitioners, 2,* 164–167.

Wagner, L., Henry, B., Giovinco, G., & Blanks, C. (1988). Suggestions for graduate education in nursing administration. *Journal of Nursing Education, 27,* 210–218.

What's happening: Survey and analysis of post-master's nurse practitioner educational programs. (1994). *Journal of the American Academy of Nurse Practitioners, 6,* 479–483.

Whitfill, K. A., & Burst, H. V. (1994). ACNM accredited and preaccredited nurse-midwifery education programs: Program Information. *Journal of Nurse Midwifery, 39,* 221–236.

Wills, E. M., & Delahoussaye, C. P. (1998). Home health graduate nursing programs in the United States. *Home Healthcare Nurse, 16*(2), 85–93.

Wood, C. M., Caldwell, M. A., Cusack, M. K., Claar-Rice, U., & Dibble, S. L. (1996). Clinical nurse specialists in California: Who claims the title? *Clinical Nurse Specialist, 10,* 283–292.

Wunderlich, G. S., Sloan, F. A., & Davis, C. K. (Eds.) (1996). *Nursing staff in hospitals and nursing homes: Is it adequate?* Washington DC: National Academy Press.

Zebelman, E. S., & Olswang, S. G. (1989). Student career goal changes during doctoral education in nursing. *Journal of Nursing Education, 28,* 53–60.

Index